The Psychology of Health and Illness

This book examines the effects of various stresses, strains, and traumas in our lives, from the womb till adulthood. The consequences of such stresses are delineated, and this book describes ways of coping with it.

Research has demonstrated, repeatedly, that chronic stress may increase unhealthy behavior which may further enhance the development of poor lifestyle habits, substance abuse, or physical inactivity. This may significantly and negatively influence not only our physical wellbeing but emotional one as well. Certain personality traits, like neuroticism for example, is positively correlated with poor physical functioning, greater alcohol consumption as well as increased cigarette smoking. Similarly, extraversion, agreeableness, and emotional stability were shown to significantly affect lifestyle, physical activity, and self-care and consequently one's health.

The chapters in this volume cover various issues that are related to and influence our health — from how adverse childhood experiences can affect our mental health, resulting in anxiety and heightened stress, to how partner violence can cause trauma on the physical and emotional health of its victims to examining the effect of assisted reproductive technology on the mother-child relationship. This book also explores the various ways to cope with the significant stress that we experience daily in our lives, as well as how self-care is important in maintaining good health and in avoiding burnout.

This book will be of great value to students, researchers, and practitioners of psychology, including health psychology and psychoanalysis. The chapters in this book were originally published in the *Journal of Psychology.*

Ami Rokach is a clinical psychologist who teaches in the Department of Psychology at York University, Toronto, Canada. He has been researching and teaching about loneliness, human sexuality, intimate relationships, and death and dying for the past 40 years.

The Psychology of Health and Illness

Edited by
Ami Rokach

Routledge
Taylor & Francis Group
LONDON AND NEW YORK

First published 2024
by Routledge
4 Park Square, Milton Park, Abingdon, Oxon, OX14 4RN

and by Routledge
605 Third Avenue, New York, NY 10158

Routledge is an imprint of the Taylor & Francis Group, an informa business

British Library Cataloguing-in-Publication Data
A catalogue record for this book is available from the British Library

ISBN13: 978-1-032-68897-8 (hbk)
ISBN13: 978-1-032-68898-5 (pbk)
ISBN13: 978-1-032-68901-2 (ebk)

DOI: 10.4324/9781032689012

Typeset in Minion Pro
by codeMantra

Publisher's Note
The publisher accepts responsibility for any inconsistencies that may have arisen during the conversion of this book from journal articles to book chapters, namely the inclusion of journal terminology.

Disclaimer
Every effort has been made to contact copyright holders for their permission to reprint material in this book. The publishers would be grateful to hear from any copyright holder who is not here acknowledged and will undertake to rectify any errors or omissions in future editions of this book.

Contents

Citation Information

The following chapters were originally published in various volumes and issues of *The Journal of Psychology*. When citing this material, please use the original page numbering for each article, as follows:

Chapter 1

Adverse Childhood Experiences (ACEs) and Help-Seeking for Health-Related Interventions in Young Adults
Canan Karatekin
The Journal of Psychology, volume 153, issue 1 (2019) pp. 6–22

Chapter 2

Intergenerational Transmission of Depression during Adolescence: The Mediating Roles of Hostile Attribution Bias, Empathic Concern, and Social Self-Concept
Xing Wei, Xi Li, Xiaoqin Teng, Jingyao Bai and Feifei Ren
The Journal of Psychology, volume 157, issue 1 (2023) pp. 13–31

Chapter 3

Contributors to Women's Perceived Stress at the Start of Assisted Reproductive Technology
Vera Skvirsky, Orit Taubman – Ben-Ari, Shirley Ben Shlomo, Joseph Azuri and Eran Horowitz
The Journal of Psychology, volume 153, issue 1 (2019) pp. 23–36

Chapter 4

Perinatal Maternal Stress and Susceptibility to Infectious Diseases in Later Childhood: An Early Life Programming Perspective
Irena Stepanikova, Elizabeth Baker, Gabriela Oates, Sanjeev Acharya, Jalal Uddin, Vojtech Thon, Jan Svancara and Lubomir Kukla
The Journal of Psychology, volume 153, issue 1 (2019) pp. 67–88

Chapter 5

Moderating Effects of Prevention-Focus on the Paths from Two Insecure Attachment Dimensions to Depression
Dong-Gwi Lee, Jae Joon Park, Byeong Hoon Bae, and Hyun-Woo Lim
The Journal of Psychology, volume 152, issue 3 (2018) pp. 151–163

Chapter 6

The Role of Mindful Self-Care in the Relationship between Emotional Intelligence and Burnout in University Students
Natasha M. Loi and Nyree Pryce
The Journal of Psychology, volume 156, issue 4 (2022) pp. 295–309

Chapter 7

The Psychology of Health and Illness: The Mental Health and Physiological Effects of Intimate Partner Violence on Women
Nancy Lutwak
The Journal of Psychology, volume 152, issue 6 (2018) pp. 373–387

Chapter 8

Emotion Regulation Difficulties Mediate the Relationship between Neuroticism and Health-Risk Behaviours in Adolescents
Parwinder Singh
The Journal of Psychology, volume 156, issue 1 (2022) pp. 48–67

Chapter 9

How Compassionate Abilities Influence the Experience of Loneliness and Quality of Life of People with and without Chronic Physical Disease?
Tânia Ramalho, Joana Pereira and Cláudia Ferreira
The Journal of Psychology, volume 155, issue 8 (2021) pp. 679–694

Chapter 10

How Future Orientation is Associated with Depressive Symptoms in Multiethnoracial Adults: Basic Psychological Needs as a Mediator
Edward C. Chang, Olivia D. Chang, Elizabeth A. Yu, Kaidi Wu, Abigael G. Lucas, P. Priscilla Lui, David Rollock, Xinjie Chen, Jameson K. Hirsch and Elizabeth L. Jeglic
The Journal of Psychology, volume 153, issue 1 (2019) pp. 89–101

Notes on Contributors

Sanjeev Acharya, Sociology Department, University of Alabama at Birmingham, USA.

Joseph Azuri, Department of Family Medicine, Tel Aviv University, Israel.

Byeong Hoon Bae, Department of Psychology, Yonsei University, Seoul, South Korea.

Jingyao Bai, Qingdao University, China.

Elizabeth Baker, Sociology Department, University of Alabama at Birmingham, USA.

Edward C. Chang, School of Social Work, University of Michigan, USA.

Olivia D. Chang, School of Social Work, University of Michigan, USA.

Xinjie Chen, Center to Support Excellence in Teaching, Stanford University, USA.

Cláudia Ferreira, Faculty of Psychology and Education Sciences, University of Coimbra, Portugal.

Jameson K. Hirsch, Department of Psychology, East Tennessee State University, Johnson City, USA.

Eran Horowitz, Faculty of Medicine, Obstetrics & Gynecology, Tel Aviv University, Israel.

Elizabeth L. Jeglic, John Jay College of Criminal Justice, CUNY, USA.

Canan Karatekin, Institute of Child Development, University of Minnesota, Minneapolis, USA.

Lubomir Kukla, Faculty of Medicine, Masaryk University, Brno, Czech Republic.

Dong-Gwi Lee, Department of Psychology, Yonsei University, Seoul, South Korea.

Xi Li, Qingdao University, China.

Hyun-Woo Lim, Department of Global Sports Industry, Hankuk University of Foreign Studies, Seoul, South Korea.

Natasha M. Loi, School of Psychology, University of New England, Australia.

Abigael G. Lucas, School of Social Work, University of Michigan, USA.

P. Priscilla Lui, Department of Psychology, Southern Methodist University, University Park, USA.

Nancy Lutwak, VA New York Harbor Healthcare System, USA.

Gabriela Oates, UAB Department of Pediatrics, University of Alabama at Birmingham, USA.

Jae Joon Park, College of Medicine, Yonsei University, Seoul, South Korea.

Joana Pereira, Faculty of Psychology and Education Sciences, University of Coimbra, Portugal.

Nyree Pryce, School of Psychology, University of New England, Australia.

Tânia Ramalho, Faculty of Psychology and Education Sciences, University of Coimbra, Portugal.

Feifei Ren, Qingdao University, China.

Ami Rokach, Department of Psychology at York University, Toronto, Canada.

David Rollock, Department of Psychological Sciences, Purdue University, USA.

Shirley Ben Shlomo, The Louis and Gabi Weisfeld School of Social Work, Bar-Ilan University, Ramat Gan, Israel.

Parwinder Singh, Department of Humanities and Social Sciences, Indian Institute of Technology Ropar, Rupnagar, India.

Vera Skvirsky, The Louis and Gabi Weisfeld School of Social Work, Bar-Ilan University, Ramat Gan, Israel.

Irena Stepanikova, Sociology Department, University of Alabama at Birmingham, USA.

Jan Svancara, Faculty of Medicine, Masaryk University, Brno, Czech Republic.

Orit Taubman – Ben-Ari, The Louis and Gabi Weisfeld School of Social Work, Bar-Ilan University, Ramat Gan, Israel.

Xiaoqin Teng, Qingdao University, China.

Vojtech Thon, Faculty of Science, Masaryk University, Brno, Czech Republic.

Jalal Uddin, Department of Community Health and Epidemiology, Dalhousie University, Halifax, Canada.

Xing Wei, Department of Psychology, Qingdao University, China.

Kaidi Wu, School of Social Work, University of Michigan, USA.

Elizabeth A. Yu, School of Social Work, University of Michigan, USA.

Introduction: Health, Illness, and the Psychological Factors Affecting Them

Ami Rokach

> Individuals who are satisfied with their lives and who experience frequent positive emotions – that is, individuals with high levels of subjective well-being … – not only feel good, but may also have reduced risk for developing coronary heart disease (CHD)… subjective well-being may buffer against the harmful health consequences of stress and exert direct influence on bodily systems, or may motivate healthy behavior.
>
> (Boehm et al., 2016; p. 1)

In this clearly formulated above quote, Boehm et al. (2016) summarized the emerging research which points out to the close links between our thoughts, emotions, behaviors and physical as well as emotional health (see also Cameron & Leventhal, 2003). Seib et al. (2014) reiterated that exposure to stressful life events, which we all experience at some points of our journey on this earth, have deleterious effects on our health and wellbeing (see Nabi et al., 2008). And while some ill health is unavoidable and some level of stress is expected in our daily lives, high level and chronic stress may increase health-compromising behavior, which may further enhance the development of poor lifestyle habits, substance abuse, or physical inactivity (Daubenmier et al., 2012). Seib et al. (2014; p. e44) further explains that "exposure to prolonged stress may change the physiological processes within the body, leading to physiological dysregulation, exacerbating proclivities for unhealthy lifestyle behaviors, and contributing to morbid health conditions" (Browning et al., 2012; Daubenmier et al., 2012).

Hershfield et al. (2013) addressed the persistent emphasis of the research literature on the effects that negative emotions have on the etiology of illness, as well as the move, lately, to examine the beneficial effects that positive emotions have on stress (Ong, 2010). However, Hershfield points, the complex interplay between positive and negative emotions in daily experience has not been well understood or researched (Davis et al., 2004). Hershfield et al. (2013) indicate that 'taking the good and the bad' in life may actually be good for us, and frequent mixed emotional experiences may actually be beneficial for one's physical health. Karademas and Tsaousis (2014) maintained, "Illness-related behavior is heavily influenced by complex processes that refer to recognizing and interpreting symptoms, understanding illness, and planning appropriate actions for coping with the disease" (p. 80). The authors examined the effect of personality and personality characteristics on mental and physical health and well-being. In that context, Karademas reviewed the Five-Factor Model (FFM), considered now the dominant framework for describing the manner in which we think, feel, and behave, pointing to five main dimensions: extraversion, agreeableness, conscientiousness, neuroticism or emotional stability, and openness to experience. Reviewing the related literature, Karademas pointed out that research indicated that high levels of neuroticism, for instance, were positively correlated with poorer physical functioning, worse illness outcomes, greater alcohol consumption as well as increased cigarette smoking (Goodwin & Stein, 2003;

Raynor & Levine, 2009). Conscientiousness was found to be a good predictor of life span mortality as well a protective factor against mortality (Taylor et al., 2009). Extraversion has been related to better health and well-being and has also been linked to health behaviors but in a diverse way (Taylor et al., 2009). Agreeableness has been shown to be related to better health behavior, while lower levels of this trait have been associated with increased mortality risk (Booth-Kewley & Vickers, 1995; see also Wiebe & Fortenberry, 2006). Shoda et al. (2002) observed that the thoughts, emotions, and behaviors that people experience are closely related to the interpersonal system of which they are a part and not just as a result of their personality alone. Shoda et al. (2002) observed that there are studies which have shown that partner personality characteristics, such as agreeableness, conscientiousness, and emotional stability, are associated with the quality of their relationship and that in turn is considered to be an important determinant of health. Similarly, people afflicted with chronic illness seem to adapt to their illness and symptoms not in isolation but while they interact and are supported by their partner (Dyrenforth et al., 2010).

As is clear from the above brief summary of some of the recent research studies, there is still quite a lot unknown and unclear indications as to the interplay of psychological and physical factors in health and illness. The present volume aimed to add to the existing literature the observations, reviews, studies, and explorations of the major 'players' in this wide field. Below is a brief summary of each of the articles included in this volume.

Karatekin examined that the effects of adverse childhood experiences (ACE), such as maltreatment, exposure to violence, and family psychopathology, are stressful and potentially traumatic events that take place during childhood. They found that students with greater exposure to early adversity were more likely than others to seek psychological/psychiatric, formal and informal types of help. Additionally, the most common reasons for seeking help were anxiety and stress in the low-ACEs group and depression in the high-ACEs group. Unfortunately, their research also demonstrated that although students with more ACEs seek more help than students with fewer ACEs, they are less likely to find these helpful and more likely to quit prematurely.

Wei, Li, Teng, Bai & Ren researched the transferring of emotionality from parents to their offspring. Their results provided evidence of cross-generational continuity in depression which is particularly prevalent during adolescence.

Svirsky, Taubman-Ben Ari, Ben Shlomo, Azuri and Horowitz examined this issue in an even earlier time of life, during assisted reproduction, for women who required it. The authors were interested in the effects of the internal resources of meaning in life, attachment style as well as self-disclosure to a woman's level of perceived stress upon commencement of Assisted Reproductive Technology (ART). Results indicated that older age, greater self-disclosure to the mother, higher perception of meaning in life, and lower anxiety attachment were related to lower levels of perceived stress. As the authors remarked, they highlighted, in their study, the importance of a woman's personal and interpersonal resources for reducing the experience of stress in the early stages of ART.

Stepanikova et al. examined perinatal maternal stress and its effects on childhood infectious diseases. The diseases that they focused on were children's diseases include eye infection, ear infection, bronchitis/lung infection, laryngitis, strep throat, cold sores, and flu/flu-like infection. They found that perinatal stress is linked to susceptibility to infectious diseases in school-age children. They reviewed that several intervention strategies to address stress in pregnant and postpartum women may benefit long-term children's health.

Lee, Park, Bae and Lim examined Korean students and what moderates the effects of prevention focus [one of Higgins's self-regulatory strategies which encompasses the motivation to obtain security, avoid undesired end states, and satisfy one's ought self], acts as a moderator of the journey from insecure attachment (attachment avoidance and attachment anxiety) to depression. They found a significant moderating effect for prevention focus on the path from attachment avoidance to depression but not on the path from attachment anxiety to depression. The authors, consequently, recommended that different interventions are needed for different combinations of persons' insecure attachment dimensions and levels of prevention focus.

Loi and Pryce looked at what contributes to academic burnout of university students. They explored the associations between emotional intelligence (EI), student well-being, mindful self-care (MSC), and academic burnout. A further aim was to investigate the mediating role of MSC in the EI-burnout relationship. Their results demonstrated that EI was positively associated with well-being and MSC and negatively associated with each dimension of academic burnout.

The next three articles addressed the quality of life, first focusing on the couple [partner violence] and then on improving the individual's satisfaction and functioning in life. ***Lutwak*** focuses on the effects of intimate partner violence, which may include PTSD, a life-altering disorder, which may also result in severely disturbed behavior by the affected victims. And as the authors asserted, survivors may require support from mental health and social service experts and even medical and pharmaceutical agents in order for them to be able to improve the quality of life, reduce depression, decrease stress, ameliorate physical symptoms, and prevent suicidal ideology. Additionally, the authors noted, there may be need for economic and employment assistance as well as placement in safe housing.

Singh examined the 'Neuroticism- Health Risk Behaviors (HRBs) adverse health' link. He examined whether emotion regulation difficulties mediates in the relationship between neuroticism and HRBs—the first two constructs of the mentioned link. The results suggested that emotion regulation difficulty may be a significant mediator in the neuroticism-HRBs link. Explaining the consequences, he noted that one's difficulty in regulating emotions might be an underlying mechanism through which high neuroticism increases the probability of indulging in HRBs, which may lead to adverse health consequences.

Ramalho, Pereira and Ferreira explored whether individuals with and without a chronic physical disease differ in levels of compassionate abilities, loneliness, and quality of life (QoL) and examined whether loneliness mediated the impact of self-compassion and of receiving compassion from others in physical, psychological, and social QoL. Results indicated that compassionate abilities have a direct effect on loneliness. The crucial role of self-compassion skills and the ability to perceive others as compassionate is highlighted in loneliness and general quality of life in both populations: those with and without a chronic physical disease.

The article by ***Chang et al.*** closes this special issue by examining the role of basic psychological needs as a mediator of the association between future orientation and depressive symptoms in a sample of multiethnoracial adults. Results indicated that the association between future orientation and depressive symptoms was accounted for by dimensions of basic psychological needs. Specifically, future orientation was negatively related to depressive symptoms through positive associations involving autonomy and competence, but not relatedness. These results suggest possible mechanisms by which believing in a changeable future might foster stronger satisfaction of basic psychological needs, especially autonomy and competence, that might help multiethnoracials garner greater protection when encountering stressful situations in their lives.

It is hoped that the research and reviews included in this volume will not only enrich readers' understanding of the field of psychology of health and illness but may be a catalyst for further research and development.

References

Boehm J. K., Chen, Y., Williams, D.R., Ryff, C.D., & Kubzansky, L.D. (2016). Subjective well-being and cardiometabolic health: An 8–11 year study of midlife adults. *Journal of Psychosomatic Research*, 85, 1–8. http://dx.doi.org/10.1016/j.jpsychores.2016.03.018.

Booth-Kewley, S., & Vickers, R.R. Jr. (1994). Associations between major domains of personality and health behavior. *Journal of Personality*, 62, 281–298.

Browning, C.R., Cagney, K.A., & Iveniuk, J. (2012). Neighborhood stressors and cardiovascular health: Crime and C-reactive protein in Dallas, USA. *Social Science & Medicine*, 75(7), 1271–1279.

Cameron, L.D., & Leventhal, H. (2003). Self-regulation, health and illness: An overview. In: L.D. Cameron & H. Leventhal H, (Eds.) *The self-regulation of health and illness behaviour* (pp. 1–13). London: Routledge.

Daubenmier, J., Lin, J., Blackburn, E., Hecht, F.M., Kristeller, J., Maninger, N., et al. (2012). Changes in stress, eating, and metabolic factors are related to changes in telomerase activity in a randomized mindfulness intervention pilot study. *Psychoneuroendocrinology*, 37(7), 917–928.

Davis, C., Zautra, A.J., & Smith, B.W. (2004). Chronic pain, stress, and the dynamics of affect differentiation. *Journal of Personality*, 72, 1133–1160. http://dx.doi.org/10.1111/j.1467-6494.2004.00293.x

Dyrenforth, P.S., Kashy, D.A., Donnellan, M.B., et al. (2010). Predicting relationship and life satisfaction from personality in nationally representative samples from three countries: The relative importance of actor, partner, and similarity effects. *Journal of Personality and Social Psychology*, 99, 690–702.

Goodwin, R.D., & Stein, M.B. (2003). Peptic ulcer disease and neuroticism in the United States adult population. *Psychotherapy and Psychosomatics*, 72, 10–15.

Hershfield, H.F., Scheibe, S.L. Sims, T., & Carstensen, L.L. (2013). When feeling bad can be good: Mixed emotions benefit physical health across adulthood. *Social Psychological and Personality Science*, 4(1), 54–61. http://dx.doi.org/10.1177/1948550612444616

Karademas, E.C., & Ioannis Tsaousis, I. (2014). The relationship of patient and spouse personality to cardiac patients' health: Two observational studies of mediation and moderation. *Annals of Behavioral Medicine*, 47, 79–91. http://dx.doi.org/10.1007/s12160-013-9523-5.

Nabi, H., Kivimaki, M., De Vogli, R., Marmot, M.G., & Singh-Manoux, A. (2008). Positive and negative affect and risk of coronary heart disease: Whitehall II prospective cohort study. *BMJ*, 337, a118.

Ong, A.D. (2010). Pathways linking positive emotion and health in later life. *Current Directions in Psychological Science*, 19, 358–362. http://dx.doi.org/10.1177/0963721410388805

Raynor D.A., & Levine H. (2009). Associations between the Five-Factor model of personality and health behaviors among college students. *Journal of American College Health*, 58, 73–82..

Seib, S., Whiteside, E., Lee, K., Humphreys, J., Dao Tran, T.H., Chopin, L., & Anderson, D. (2014). Stress, lifestyle, and quality of life in midlife and older Australian women: Results from the stress and the health of women study. *Women's Health Issues*, 24(1), e43–e52. http://dx.doi.org/10.1016/j.whi.2013.11.004.

Shoda, Y., LeeTierman, S., & Mischel, W. (2002). Personality as a dynamic system: Emergence of stability and distinctiveness from intra- and interpersonal interactions. *Personality and Social Psychology Review*, 6, 316–325.

Taylor, M.D., Whiteman, M.C., Fowkes, G.R., et al. (2009). Five Factor Model personality traits and all-cause mortality in the Edinburgh Artery Study Cohort. *Psychosomatic Medicine*, 71, 631–641.

Wiebe, D.J., & Fortenberry, K.T. (2006). Mechanisms relating personality and health. In: M.E. Vollrath (Ed). *Handbook of personality and health* (pp. 137–156). Chichester: Wiley.

Adverse Childhood Experiences (ACEs) and Help-Seeking for Health-Related Interventions in Young Adults

Canan Karatekin

ABSTRACT

Although college students have increasingly higher health needs, they underutilize interventions. Given the association between adverse childhood experiences (ACEs) and poor health, the goal of this study was to examine the contribution of ACEs in undergraduates to seeking help for problems related to health. An online survey of students ($N = 321$, 76% female, 72% Caucasian) in a large public university showed that respondents with more ACEs were more likely to seek help, including both professional and informal types of help. However, they were less likely to find interventions helpful and more likely to quit prematurely. Common reasons for seeking help were anxiety, stress, and depression, with depression more prevalent in the high-ACEs group. More ACEs were associated with more unmet needs and greater likelihood of obtaining health information from school, another professional, or the media. More research is needed on how to harness the power of informal sources of help to improve the health of students with more ACEs, how to tailor health-related messages to fit their needs, and why students with more ACEs find interventions less helpful. Finally results suggest that ACEs shape not only lifelong health but also behaviors related to seeking help in young adults.

Three quarters of lifelong mental disorders emerge by age 24 (Kessler et al., 2005), and college students have increasingly higher and persistent health needs (Bonnie, Stroud, & Breiner, 2015; Eagan et al., 2014; Gallagher, 2014; Hunt & Eisenberg, 2010). Yet, research consistently shows that college students underutilize interventions (Castillo & Schwartz, 2013; Herman et al., 2011; Hunt & Eisenberg, 2010). The goal of the current study was to examine whether adverse childhood experiences (ACEs) play a role in patterns of seeking help for health problems in young adults attending college.

ACEs, such as maltreatment, exposure to violence, and family psychopathology, are stressful and potentially traumatic events that take place during childhood (Felitti et al., 1998). Over a third of adults in the U.S. have been exposed to at least two ACEs (Bynum et al., 2010), and recent cohorts report more ACEs than older cohorts (Austin & Herrick, 2014; Bynum et al., 2010; Logan-Greene, Green, Nurius, & Longhi, 2014).

ACEs have emerged as a significant factor in public health. A large body of research shows robust associations between ACEs and many mental and physical health outcomes, physiological indicators of future health status, and premature mortality (Larkin, Shields, & Anda, 2012).

College students have high lifetime rates of maltreatment (Berzenski & Yates, 2011) and other potentially traumatic events (Read, Ouimette, White, Colder, & Farrow, 2011). There is little peer-reviewed research on ACEs in college students, although almost 70% of all 18- to 19-year-olds in the U.S. enroll in college ("Mobile Digest of Education Statistics, 2013"). The one study to examine childhood adversities in college students, in Ireland, found that 35% had at least two ACEs (McGavock & Spratt, 2014). Another study, conducted in the 1990s in the U.S., found 38–53% of college students had at least two *lifetime* adverse events (Smyth, Hockemeyer, Heron, Wonderlich, & Pennebaker, 2008). An annual survey of health in University of Minnesota students included ACEs for the first time in Spring 2015 and found that almost 60% reported having experienced two or more ACEs (Boynton Health Service, 2015).

One factor contributing to increasing mental health problems in college students may be increasing burden of ACEs. However, no study has examined the contribution of ACEs to the health of college students or to their patterns of seeking help. The current study is part of a larger study of health and ACEs in college students. In a previous paper (author names withheld, 2016), we showed that despite having parents with high levels of education and feeling high levels of social support, students reported a high level of mental health problems and ACEs rates similar to those in the State's general population. Those with more ACEs experienced more stress and less social support, and ACEs, social support, and stress explained over half the variance in mental health scores. In a second paper (author names withheld, 2018), we demonstrated that students with more ACEs were less likely to take active charge of their own health and to be more concerned with preventing negative outcomes than promoting positive outcomes, which may have implications for framing messages about health-related interventions for students with more ACEs.

The current paper focuses on the help-seeking behavior of college students as a function of ACEs. As there is no research on this question, the goal of this exploratory study was to generate ideas for hypothesis-driven research. The following questions were addressed:

1. Do students with fewer versus more ACEs differ in the types of help they seek? Studies of college students seeking help have focused almost exclusively on formal psychological types of help, such as individual therapy or counseling (e.g., Gallagher, 2014). However, ACEs have been associated with both mental and physical problems (Larkin et al., 2012), and it is important not to ignore the close connection between mental and physical health. In addition, studies of seeking help in individuals with ACEs often focus on archival data based on health care utilization (Larkin et al., 2012). Yet, individuals may utilize informal types of help (e.g., self-help groups) to a greater extent than formal types of help (Goldstrom et al., 2006). Thus, we used a broad definition of help.
2. Do students with more versus fewer ACEs differ in the extent to which they find interventions helpful? There are only a few studies on the evaluation of

intervention outcomes for individuals with ACEs (Nemeroff et al., 2003) or perceptions of college students regarding the help they receive. One study found that only two-thirds of the students reported that counseling helped them with their academic performance (Gallagher, 2014).

3. Do students with fewer versus more ACEs differ in the kinds of problems they are and are not seeking help for? College students show high levels of anxiety, depression, and substance use (Blanco et al., 2008; Eagan et al., 2014; Eisenberg, Golberstein, & Gollust, 2007; Gallagher, 2014; Hunt & Eisenberg, 2010). However, physical problems are not assessed or are covered minimally in this research, and neither studies on ACEs nor on students focus as much on health problems students are *not* seeking help for. Yet, information on unmet health needs is crucial for designing effective interventions to meet the needs of this population.
4. Do ACEs make a difference in where students obtain information regarding interventions related to health? The answer has implications for dissemination of information regarding interventions. Yet, there is almost no research on this topic in either the literature on ACEs or on mental health in college students. One exception is a study that examined sources college students use to obtain information related to health (American College Health Association-National College Health Assessment Spring 2008 Reference Group Data Report (Abridged): The American College Health Association, 2009). The Internet, family, friends, and health center medical staffs were the most frequently sought sources.

Method

Participants

Participants were undergraduates at a large public Midwestern university, recruited through Psychology classes offering course credit for research participation. The sample consisted of 321 students (76% female, 23% male, 1% "other"), with a median age of 19.0 ($M = 20.1$, $SD = 3.1$). Although the ages of the participants ranged from 18 to 49, 97% of the samples were between 18 and 25. The sample was divided among freshmen (32%), sophomores (28%), juniors (19%), and seniors (20%). Participants were predominantly Caucasian (71%), followed by Asian (20%), and African–American (3%), and those self-identifying as multiracial (3%), "other" (2%), or Native American (0.3%). Only 2% identified as Hispanic. Some students (16%) were born outside the U.S.; most (69%) were Asians.

Procedure

Participants responded to a questionnaire through a secure online survey service (Qualtrics). They received course credit for completing the survey, which was estimated to take at most 1½ hours. This manuscript includes data from a subset of the measures. The study was approved by the University's Institutional Review Board.

Measures

Parental Education

There is no established measure of childhood socioeconomic status (SES), and controversy rages regarding measures of childhood SES and their reliability and validity (Braveman et al., 2005). We assessed parental education as a proxy for childhood SES. Participants rated the highest grade completed by their parents or primary caretakers from 1 (no formal education) to 7 (completed post-college work), with options for "don't know" and "no primary male/female caretaker." Parents' average score was calculated; if information was provided for only one parent, that parent's level of education was used.

ACEs

Although the original ACEs questionnaire (Felitti et al., 1998) covers important adversities, its psychometric properties have not been established and it has been criticized for omitting essential areas of adversity (Finkelhor, Shattuck, Turner, & Hamby, 2013). Therefore, we adapted the validated Juvenile Victimization Questionnaire (JVQ) (Finkelhor et al., 2013) by adding questions from the original ACEs questionnaire and slightly editing the wording to be appropriate for adults. This 33-item instrument covered nine domains of moderate to severe adversity between ages 0 and 18: child maltreatment, household dysfunction, separation from parental figures, peer and sibling victimization, discrimination, exposure to community violence, property victimization, bad accident or illness of someone close, and social isolation. Participants responded to each question with a "yes" or "no"; "yes" responses were summed to yield an ACEs score that could range from 0 to 33. The measure had good internal consistency in the current sample (Cronbach's alpha = .86).

Interventions

As there is no established questionnaire that covers utilization of both formal and informal types of help for both mental and physical problems, a questionnaire was created for this study. Participants were asked "Have you received any of the following types of help for health-related problems *in the past two years*? Please respond yes or no for all items that apply. This question does *not* apply to one-time visits, such as a visit to a health care professional for an acute condition (e.g., a visit to urgent care or an emergency department), a preventive visit (e.g., to get a flu shot), or a one-time visit to a massage therapist, etc." They were provided with a list of 32 types of interventions (Table 1). A 2-year limit was chosen to minimize memory limitations. Interventions were divided into medical versus psychological/psychiatric on one hand, and formal versus informal on the other hand (indicated in Table 1).

For each intervention endorsed, students were asked: "What was the reason why you sought this help, in about five words or less (e.g., dizziness, depression, stress, mourning a loss, relationship problems, broken bone, etc.)?" Next, they responded with a "yes" or "no" to the question "Did you stop prematurely, before the problem you sought help

Table 1. Percent of Students in the Low- and High-ACEs Groups Who Indicated using Different Kinds of Help.

	Low ACEs ($N = 171$)	High ACEs ($N = 150$)
Hospitalizations, partial hospitalization, or day treatment program for medical problems (M, F)	11	20
Hospitalizations, partial hospitalizations, or day treatment program for psychological or psychiatric problems (P, F)	2	7
Hospitalizations, partial hospitalizations, day treatment, or rehab for drug or alcohol use problems (P, F)	1	5
Individual outpatient visits with a general practitioner to address medical problems (e.g., someone in family practice, nurse, GP, etc.) (M, F)	19	32
Individual outpatient visits with a medical specialist to address medical problems (e.g., a neurologist; oncologist; ear, nose and throat specialist, etc.) (M, F)	19	24
Physical therapy (M, F)	18	21
Occupational therapy (F)	0	3
Massage therapy (F)	14	17
Meetings with a nutritionist (M, F)	5	9
Group activities for improving physical health (e.g., organized physical fitness activities, zumba classes, yoga classes, etc.) (M, F)	40	36
Individual outpatient visits with a psychologist, social worker, or psychiatrist for psychosocial interventions (e.g., cognitive-behavior therapy, psychodynamic therapy, mindfulness, general talk therapy, etc.) (P, F)	16	28
Individual outpatient visits with a psychiatrist for management of medications related to psychological or psychiatric problems (e.g., medications for ADHD, depression, anxiety, etc.) (P, F)	9	19
Interventions with a broad focus, led by a professional (i.e., interventions that involved active participation by you, your teachers, your family, friends, other people working with you or in your community, etc.) (P, F)	1	3
Formal group-based treatments for psychological problems (i.e., group therapy for eating disorders) (P, F)	3	7
Workshops for psychological problems, by a professional (e.g., a workshop on mindfulness or healthy living) (P, F)	3	5
Workshops for medical problems, led by a professional (e.g., a workshop on how to live with diabetes) (M, F)	0	3
Family therapy by a professional (e.g., psychologist, social worker, etc.) (P, F)	1	4
Couples therapy by a professional (e.g.,. psychologist, social worker, etc.) (P, F)	0	4
Ongoing sessions with a neuropsychologist (e.g., for cognitive rehabilitation) (P, F)	0	3
Life coaching (P, F)	4	3
Alternative medicine on a one-on-one basis (e.g., homeopathy, acupuncture, Ayurvedic medicine) (M, Inf)	7	4
Informal group-based interventions for a psychological problem (e.g., support groups in the community, such as Alcoholics Anonymous; other groups getting together on their own around a mental health issue) (P, Inf)	0	7
Informal group-based interventions for a medical problem (e.g., support groups in the community around a physical health issue) (M, Inf)	1	1
Informal support from friends and relatives (P, Inf)	37	47
Informal support from religious authorities or organizations (P, Inf)	9	12
Online self-guided interventions for psychological issues (e.g., online course on stress management or brain training exercises) (P, Inf)	4	13
Online support groups/chat rooms around a mental health issue (P, Inf)	1	5

(continued)

Table 1. Continued.

	Low ACEs ($N = 171$)	High ACEs ($N = 150$)
Online support groups/chat rooms around a medical issue (M, Inf)	2	3
Other personally administered interventions related to psychological problems (e.g., self-help books related to mental health; over-the-counter medications such as St. John's wort) (P, Inf)	8	18
Other personally administered interventions related to medical problems (e.g., self-help books related to health; over-the-counter medications) (M, Inf)	9	16
Accommodations for medical or physical disabilities (e.g., extra time on exams) (M, F)	4	4
Accommodations for psychological problems (e.g., extra time on exams) (P, F)	5	10
Other	1	1

Participants were asked to check all responses that applied, so percentages do not add up to 100. M: Help focused on medical or physical issues; P: Help focused on psychological or psychiatric issues; F: Formal help by a qualified or professional provider; Inf: Informal help.

for was resolved? For example, did you stop receiving this help before a predetermined number of sessions/visits or before the person helping you said you were ready to stop?" Finally, they rated how helpful the intervention was, from 1 ("extremely unhelpful") to 10 ("extremely helpful").

Unmet Health Needs

Participants were asked: "Are there any mental or physical health problems that are *currently* bothering you for which you have *not* sought any help? Please check all items that apply. If you are not sure about the category, please write the name of the problem at the end of this section." As there is no established measure for assessing a broad range of unmet mental and physical health needs, ICD-9 (World Health Organization, 1978) categories were used for medical problems, with examples for each category, and DSM-V (American Psychiatric Association, 2013) codes were used for psychiatric problems. Several other problems with lifestyle and relationships were added. All conditions are listed in Table 2.

Sources of Information

Participants were asked "If you have sought help for *health-related problems* in the past two years, where did you find out about this help? Please check all that apply." Response options were: (1) Google and other search engines; (2) General information distributed by the university (e.g., brochures, websites, workshops); (3) Information I learned in my classes and from my teachers; (4) Referral by another professional, (5) Recommendations of friends and family, (6) Facebook, Twitter, and other social networking sites, (7) Movies & TV shows; (8) Other media (TV or radio news, news sources on the internet, like cnn.com, etc.; popular magazines, e.g., *People*); (9) Self-help books; (10) Other.

Table 2. Percent of Students Indicating They Currently had Conditions They Were not Seeking Help for.

	Low ACEs ($N = 171$)	High ACEs ($N = 150$)
Categories from ICD-9		
Infectious and parasitic diseases, not including colds or flu	2	2
Neoplasms	0	0
Endocrine, nutritional, and metabolic diseases, immunity disorders	1	6
Diseases of the blood and blood-forming organs	0	2
Diseases of the nervous system and sense organs	1	2
Diseases of the circulatory system	1	1
Diseases of the respiratory system	3	4
Diseases of the digestive system	2	4
Diseases of the genitourinary system	1	3
Diseases of the skin and subcutaneous tissue	7	8
Diseases of the musculoskeletal system and connective tissue	1	1
Categories from DSM-V		
Communication disorders	1	0
Autism spectrum disorder	0	1
ADHD or ADD	3	5
Learning disorders or disabilities	1	1
Motor disorders	0	0
Schizophrenia spectrum and other psychotic disorders	0	1
Bipolar and related disorders	2	2
Depressive disorders	6	21
Anxiety disorders	7	22
Obsessive-compulsive and related disorders	2	4
Trauma and stressor-related disorders	0	4
Dissociative disorders	0	1
Somatic symptom and related disorders	0	0
Eating disorders	4	9
Sleep/wake disorders	2	6
Problems related to sexual functioning	1	5
Gender dysphoria	0	1
Disruptive, impulse control, and conduct disorders	0	0
Substance-related and addictive disorders	2	3
Personality disorders	0	3
Issues related to lifestyle and relationships		
Stress	21	40
Poor lifestyle (e.g., diet, exercise)	5	20
Interactions with family	1	11
Interactions with peers	3	8
Interactions with romantic partners	2	11
Sexual victimization	1	1
Other	3	2

Participants were asked to indicate all responses that applied; thus, the percentages do not add up to 100.

Data Analyses

Data were checked for missing values, frequencies, minima, and maxima, and continuous data were checked for outliers and deviations from normality. No outliers were found. If data were not normally distributed, the Box-Cox procedure was used to determine the most appropriate transformation. Total number of types of interventions was transformed by taking its natural logarithm. For group comparisons, students were divided into low- and high-ACEs groups based on a median split ($Mdn = 3$). There were 171 students (53%) with 0 to 2 ACEs and 150 students with 3 or more ACEs (47%). However, the more sensitive continuous measure of ACEs was used whenever possible. Linear regressions were used to analyze continuous outcomes, and logistic regressions to analyze dichotomous outcomes. Parental education and gender were used as covariates in all regression analyses. Significance levels were set at .05. Bonferroni's corrections were used when multiple tests were conducted on measures where responses were not independent of each other (e.g., types of help sought).

Word clouds were created for the open-ended question regarding the reasons why students sought the types of help they did. First, the words were checked for spelling and consistency (e.g., "bipolar," "not bi-polar"). Common words (e.g., "I", "to," and "and"), and responses that did not answer the question (e.g., "no reason") were removed. Similar reasons that were worded slightly differently were standardized (e.g., "to stay fit," and "to stay in shape" were changed to "fitness", and "anxiety in school" and "medications for anxiety" were changed to "anxiety"). A minimum frequency of two was set for the words to be included in the word cloud. All analyses were conducted in R, Version 3.4.4 (R Core Team, 2017).

Results

Types of Help Sought

Most (77%; $N = 321$) students indicated that they had sought at least one form of help. In the preceding two years, students in the low-ACEs group had sought a median of two types of help ($M = 2.5$, $SD = 2.6$), whereas students in the high-ACEs group had sought a median of three types of help ($M = 3.9$, $SD = 4.1$). Group differences in types of help can be observed almost across the board (Table 1), although the magnitude of the difference varied across interventions. A linear regression indicated that, after controlling for parental education and gender, the more ACEs students had been exposed to, the more types of help they had sought, t (314) = 6.02, $p < .001$, B = 0.06 (CI = .04–.07), SE = 0.01, $\beta = .32$.

Four logistic regressions were conducted, with Bonferroni's correction, to examine differences between ACE groups in types of help sought (note that types of help were not mutually exclusive). Higher numbers of ACEs were associated with greater likelihood of having sought help for psychological/psychiatric issues, z (314) = 4.36, $p < .001$, B = 0.15, SE = .03, OR = 1.16 (CI = 1.09–1.24), formal types of help, z (314) = 2.76, $p = .006$, B = 0.10, SE = .04, OR = 1.10 (CI = 1.03–1.18), and informal types of help, z (314) = 3.00, $p = .003$, B = 0.08, SE = .03, OR = 1.09 (CI = 1.03–1.15). With the Bonferroni correction, the effect just missed significance for help around medical/physical issues, $p = .021$.

Perceived Helpfulness of the Interventions

Increasing numbers of ACEs were associated with decreasing ratings of the helpfulness of the interventions, t (239) = −3.54, $p < .001$, B = −0.08 (CI = −0.13– −.04), SE = .02, $\beta = -.22$. A third (30%) of the high-ACEs students indicated that they had stopped the intervention prematurely, compared to only 16% of the low-ACEs students. More ACEs were associated with a greater likelihood of stopping interventions prematurely, z (314) = 4.90, $p < .001$, B = 0.15, SE = 0.03, OR = 1.16 (CI = 1.09–1.23).

Reasons for Seeking Help

Depression, stress, and anxiety dominated the stated reasons for seeking help in both groups (Figure 1). In the high-ACEs group, "depression," "stress," "anxiety" were used 95, 79, and 56 times, respectively. In the low-ACEs group, the corresponding counts were 23, 47, and 39.

Problems for Which Participants Were not Seeking Help

Half (50%, $N = 161$) the participants reported that they had conditions they were currently suffering from that they had not sought help for (Table 2). Students with high levels of ACEs had more unmet needs, with the greatest differences in depression, anxiety, stress, lifestyle, and family interactions (Table 2). In the high-ACEs group, 67% indicated there was a problem they were not seeking help for. In the low-ACEs group, the proportion was only 37%. A higher number of ACEs was associated with a higher

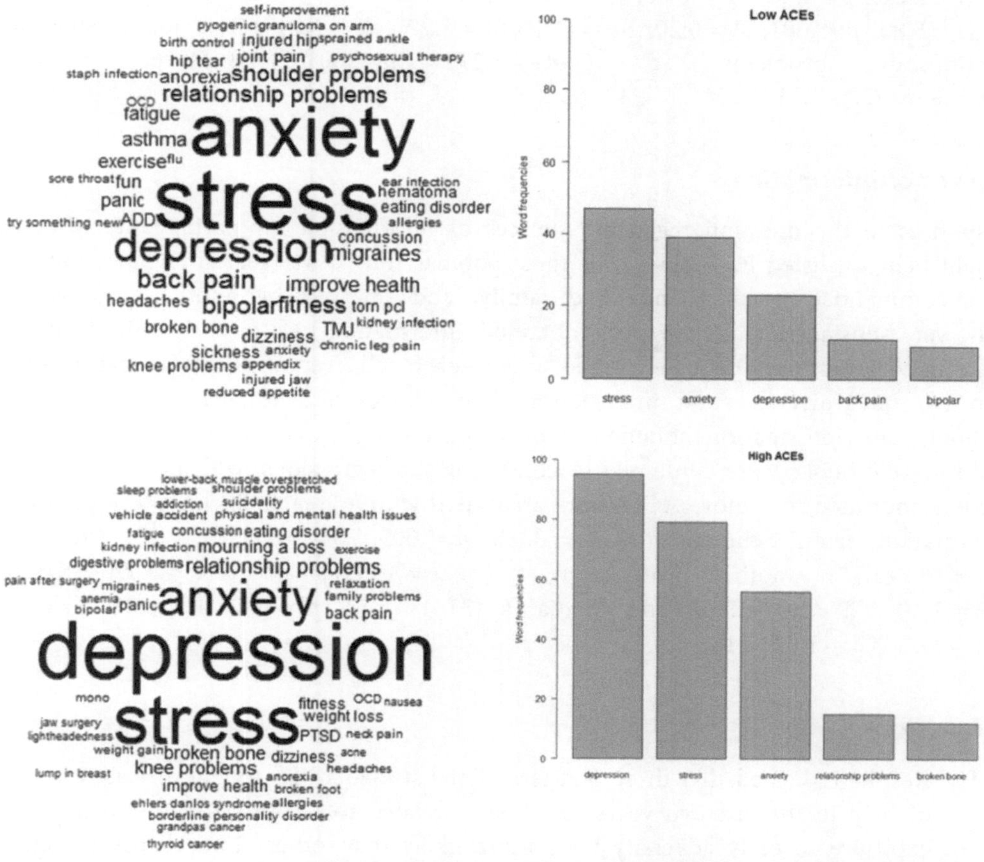

Figure 1. Word cloud figures of reasons why students sought the types of help they did in the (a) low-ACEs ($N = 171$) and (c) high-ACEs ($N = 150$) groups, and bar plots of the five most frequent reasons in the (b) low-ACEs and (d) high-ACEs groups.

Table 3. Percentages of Students Indicating Which Sources of Information They Used about Problems Related to Health.

	Low ACEs ($N = 171$)	High ACEs ($N = 150$)
Google and other search engines	45	54
Recommendations of friends and family	33	35
Referral by another professional	27	37
General information distributed by the university	14	25
Information learned in classes and from teachers	12	25
Facebook, Twitter, and other social networking sites	5	11
Movies and TV shows	3	7
Other media (TV or radio news, news sources on the internet, popular magazines)	2	9
Self-help books	2	6
Other	3	4

Participants were asked to indicate all responses that applied; thus, the percentages do not add up to 100.

likelihood of having a problem that the student was not seeking help for, z (314) = 5.83, $p < .001$, B = 0.21, SE = .04, OR = 1.25 (CI = 1.16–1.35).

Logistic regressions, with Bonferroni's correction, indicated that the more ACEs students had, the more unmet needs they were likely to have in terms of medical, z (314) = 2.62, $p = .009$, B = 0.08, SE = .03, OR = 1.08 (CI = 1.02–1.15), psychiatric, z (314) = 5.80, $p < .001$, B = 0.20, SE = .03, OR = 1.22 (CI = 1.14–1.31), and lifestyle and relationship problems, z (314) = 5.29, $p < .001$, B = 0.16, SE = .03, OR = 1.18 (CI = 1.11–1.25).

Sources of Information

Responses to the question regarding sources of information for participants who had sought help are listed in Table 3. The most popular source was search engines, followed by recommendations of friends and family, and referrals by another professional. However, substantial numbers also obtained information related to health from the University. To ensure adequate sample sizes in each cell, responses for general information by the University and information from classes and teachers were combined (School), and information obtained from social media, movies and TV, other media, and self-help books were combined (Media). Logistic regressions, with Bonferroni's correction, indicated that more ACEs were associated with a greater likelihood of obtaining information from School, z (314) = 3.02, $p = .003$, B = 0.08, SE = .03, OR = 1.09 (CI = 1.03–1.15), another professional, z (311) = 3.45, $p = .001$, B = 0.09, SE = .03, OR = 1.10 (CI = 1.04–1.16), and Media, z (314) = 2.72, $p = .007$, B = 0.08, SE = .03, OR = 1.09 (CI = 1.02–1.16).

Discussion

1. Results indicated that three quarters of the students had sought at least one type of help in the last two years for reasons related to health. Students with greater exposure to early adversity were more likely than others to seek psychological/psychiatric, formal and informal types of help. Group differences in seeking help for medical conditions just missed significance, and the relatively smaller effect may be attributable to the relatively young age of the sample.

Results are consistent with other research indicating that college students have extensive health needs (Bonnie et al., 2015; Eagan et al., 2014; Gallagher, 2014; Hunt & Eisenberg, 2010). However, contrary to previous research on under-utilization of help in college students (Castillo & Schwartz, 2013; Herman et al., 2011; Hunt & Eisenberg, 2010), current findings demonstrate that students do utilize many types of interventions for their health problems. The discrepancy is likely due to the narrow definition of health care utilization in previous studies. There is no established taxonomy of types of help individuals seek for health problems; however, studies on utilization of health care in college students (Herman et al., 2011; Hunt & Eisenberg, 2010) or in individuals who have been maltreated or exposed to early adversity (Björkenstam et al., 2013; Chartier, Walker, & Naimark, 2010) often focus on formal, professional types of help. Yet, in the mental health field, for example, peer-to-peer interventions have been estimated to outnumber traditional forms of intervention methods by almost 2 to 1 (Goldstrom et al., 2006). Current results suggest that ignoring non-professional types of help will underestimate the true extent of help-seeking and potential interactions among different types of help.

Given the high prevalence of psychological/psychiatric problems associated with ACEs in both adolescence and adulthood (Austin & Herrick, 2014; Larkin et al., 2012; McLaughlin et al., 2012) and high levels of health care utilization in this population (Chartier et al., 2010), it is not surprising that students with more ACEs are more likely to seek help around these issues. Current findings contribute to the ACEs literature by further demonstrating that they are also more likely to seek informal types of help. More research is needed on why this may be the case, on whether informal types of help may be beneficial or detrimental to their health, and on how to harness the power of these forms of help to improve their health. For example, previous studies indicate that peers are at least as effective as professionals in providing certain kinds of help for health problems, cost less, and are especially good at reaching low-income, less educated, and minority individuals (Cook et al., 2012; Day, Michelson, Thomson, Penney, & Draper, 2012; Tang, Funnell, Gillard, Nwankwo, & Heisler, 2011; Webel, Okonsky, Trompeta, & Holzemer, 2010). Peer-to-peer interventions are recommended by the federal government (Campbell & Leaver, 2003; Frese, Knight, & Saks, 2009), Veterans' Administration (Davidson, Chinman, Sells, & Rowe, 2005), World Health Organization (Bronner, Barber, & Davis, 2001), American Cancer Society (Campbell, Phaneuf, & Deane, 2004), and National Alliance on Mental Illness (n.d.), and increasingly reimbursed by Medicare/Medicaid and insurance companies as evidence-based practices (Ahmed et al., 2012; Daniels et al., 2013).

Current findings also indicate that ACEs account for at least some of the variability in the extent to which college students seek help for problems related to their health. This knowledge can be helpful in tailoring interventions that are better suited to college students' needs.

2. Although students with more ACEs seek more help than students with fewer ACEs, they are less likely to find these helpful and more likely to quit prematurely. This result echoes the original observation that gave rise to research on

ACEs, which showed that individuals with a history of emotional trauma and household dysfunction had elevated rates of drop out (Felitti & Anda, 2010) and were less likely to maintain their weight loss in a program for morbidly obese individuals (Felitti & Williams, 1998). More research is needed on why individuals with more ACEs are less satisfied or less likely to follow through with the help they receive, as negative experiences may discourage them from seeking further help. This pattern of seeking help is likely to be cost-ineffective from both a personal and societal point of view. The interventions they seek may not be as effective, perhaps because they are not based on evidence or tailored to the needs of individuals with ACEs, or because they do not seek the right type of intervention. Characteristics associated with high levels of ACEs (e.g., higher stress levels, poorer interpersonal skills, less self-efficacy) may also render interventions less effective for them (Kendall-Tackett, 2002). More research is needed on evaluation of outcomes and subjective perceptions of effectiveness as a function of level of ACEs and the factors that contribute to the ineffectiveness of interventions. Current results also suggest that one aspect of the developmental cascade that leads to poor health in individuals with ACEs may be the ineffectiveness of interventions utilized by these individuals.

3. The most common reasons for seeking help were anxiety and stress in the low-ACEs group and depression in the high-ACEs group. These concerns are consistent with previous studies of college students (Blanco et al., 2008; Eagan et al., 2014; Eisenberg et al., 2007; Gallagher, 2014; Hunt & Eisenberg, 2010), although current results demonstrate that their proportions differ as a function of ACEs. The conditions that students were *not* seeking help for also included depression, anxiety, stress, as well as lifestyle and family interactions, which are likely interrelated. Students with more ACEs were more likely to have unmet needs, including medical, psychiatric, and lifestyle/relationship problems. Results have implications for designing medical and psychological interventions for individuals with more ACEs, as unmet health needs can interfere with the success of interventions that they do seek help for. These unmet needs can also lead to the kinds of dysfunctional coping mechanisms and health-risk behaviors hypothesized to mediate the relationship between ACEs and poor health (Bellis et al., 2014; Felitti et al., 1998; Kendall-Tackett, 2002).
4. Most students indicated that they obtained their information about interventions related to health from search engines, followed by referrals from friends, family, and professionals. These results are highly consistent with the only previous study that examined sources of students' information about health ("American College Health Association-National College Health Assessment Spring 2008 Reference Group Data Report (Abridged)," 2009). Furthermore, students with more ACEs were more likely to obtain their information from school, another professional, or the media compared to students with fewer ACEs. Despite the dangers of self-diagnosis on the Internet, these results can be viewed as opportunities for disseminating information about interventions related to health. In particular, the fact that students with more ACEs are more likely to obtain information from university-provided resources provides a valuable opportunity for schools to reach out to at-risk students.

Limitations

Data are based on a convenience sample from a single university. However, mental health problems in young adults have not been found to differ as a function of the type of university (Eisenberg et al., 2007). Second, data were based on self-report. Nevertheless, if archival or more objective data had been used, results would have missed group differences in utilization of informal forms of help as well as unmet health needs. Third, the psychometric properties of the questionnaires have not been established. It is hoped that the current results can form a basis for more psychometrically sound measures. A manuscript on the psychometric properties of the ACEs questionnaire used in the current study in approximately 1500 students in the same university is currently in preparation. Finally, ACEs were assessed retrospectively. However, comparisons of prospective and retrospective data show no bias in assessment and no differences among associations between number of ACEs and outcomes as a function of time of reporting (Hardt, Vellaisamy, & Schoon, 2010). The young age of these participants ($Mdn = 19$) should have also minimized bias due to memory limitations.

Summary and Conclusions

On the one hand, there is a very large body of research demonstrating a strong association between ACEs and poor health outcomes throughout life, despite higher rates of health care utilization. Yet, there is little research on the full extent of help that individuals with ACEs receive, how effectively they utilize this help, and what schools can do to address these needs. On the other hand, colleges are having a difficult time addressing the increasingly higher health needs of their students. Yet, there is almost no research on the contribution of ACEs to these health problems and how research on ACEs can be used to improve students' well-being.

The current study combined these strands of research by examining the contribution of ACEs to the health of college students and their proclivity to seek help for their health problems. Compared to students with fewer ACEs, students with more ACEs had sought more types of help, including psychological/psychiatric, formal and informal types of help. They were more likely to seek help for depression, as well as anxiety and stress, but also more likely to still have unmet needs in terms of depression, anxiety, stress, lifestyle and family interactions. They were also more likely to find the "interventions" unhelpful and to quit prematurely. Finally, they were more likely to obtain their health-related information from university sources, another professional, and the media.

Results suggest that colleges need to pay attention to students' history of ACEs need to serve them better. Results further suggest that both researchers and health care providers need to take into account informal, non-professional sources of help that individuals are utilizing to cope with their health problems and take advantage of these sources of help to improve health. Findings also suggest that researchers should give more emphasis to understanding individuals' perceptions of formal and informal types of help as less satisfactory in uncovering the mediators of the relationship between ACEs and poor health.

Finally, results suggest that it may be fruitful to conceptualize a high number of ACEs as a coherent condition characterized by an accumulation of risk factors that shapes not only lifelong health trajectories but also attitudes toward health and seeking help even in young adults. ACEs need to be taken into consideration in young adults' health needs and in the design, implementation, and dissemination of interventions related to health for this population.

Acknowledgments

The author would like to thank Tori Simenec for her help with administering the survey, and Brandon Almy and Michael Kim for their comments on the paper.

Disclosure statement

The author has no conflicts of interest and was not paid to write this manuscript.

References

Ahmed, A. O., Doane, N. J., Mabe, P. A., Buckley, P. F., Birgenheir, D., & Goodrum, N. M. (2012). Peers and peer-led interventions for people with schizophrenia. *Psychiatric Clinics of North America*, *35*, 699–715. doi:10.1016/j.psc.2012.06.009

American College Health Association-National College Health Assessment Spring 2008 Reference Group Data Report (Abridged): The American College Health Association. (2009). American College Health Association-National College Health Assessment Spring 2008 Reference Group Data Report (Abridged): The American College Health Association. *Journal of American College Health*, *57*, 477–488. doi:10.3200/JACH.57.5.477-488

American Psychiatric Association. (2013). *Diagnostic and statistical manual of mental disorders (DSM, 5 ®)*. Washington, DC.: American Psychiatric Association.

Austin, A., E., & Herrick, H., W. (2014). *The effect of adverse childhood experiences on adult health: 2012 North Carolina Behavioral Risk Factor Surveillance System Survey. (No. (SCHS Study No. 167))*. Raleigh: North Carolina Department of Health and Human Services, Division of Public Health.

Bellis, M. A., Hughes, K., Leckenby, N., Jones, L., Baban, A., Kachaeva, M., … Terzic, N. (2014). Adverse childhood experiences and associations with health-harming behaviours in young adults: Surveys in eight eastern European countries. *Bulletin of the World Health Organization*, *92*, 641–655. doi:10.2471/BLT.13.129247

Berzenski, S. R., & Yates, T. M. (2011). Classes and consequences of multiple maltreatment: A person-centered analysis. *Child Maltreatment*, *16*, 250–261. doi:10.1177/1077559511428353

Björkenstam, E., Hjern, A., Mittendorfer-Rutz, E., Vinnerljung, B., Hallqvist, J., & Ljung, R. (2013). Multi-exposure and clustering of adverse childhood experiences, socioeconomic differences and psychotropic medication in young adults. *PLoS ONE*, *8*, e53551. doi:10.1371/journal.pone.0053551

Blanco, C., Okuda, M., Wright, C., Hasin, D. S., Grant, B. F., Liu, S.-M., & Olfson, M. (2008). Mental health of college students and their non-college-attending peers: Results from the National Epidemiologic Study on Alcohol and Related Conditions. *Archives of General Psychiatry, 65*, 1429–1437. doi:10.1001/archpsyc.65.12.1429

Bonnie, R. J., Stroud, C., & Breiner, H. (Eds.). (2015). *Investing in the health and well-being of young adults*. Washington, D.C.: National Academies Press.

Boynton Health Service Survey Team. (2015). *2015 College Student Health Survey Report*. Retrieved from. https://boynton.umn.edu/sites/boynton.umn.edu/files/2018-02/MNPostsecondaryStudents_CSHSReport_2015.pdf

Braveman, P. A., Cubbin, C., Egerter, S., Chideya, S., Marchi, K. S., Metzler, M., & Posner, S. (2005). Socioeconomic status in health research: One size does not fit all. *JAMA, 294*, 2879–2888. doi:10.1001/jama.294.22.2879

Bronner, Y., Barber, T., & Davis, S. (2001). Breastfeeding peer counseling: Policy implications. *Journal of Human Lactation, 17*, 105–109. doi:10.1177/089033440101700203

Bynum, L., Griffin, T., Riding, D. L., Wynkoop, K. S., Anda, R. F., Edwards, V. J., … Croft, J. B. (2010). Adverse childhood experiences reported by adults—Five states, 2009. *Morbidity and Mortality Weekly Report, 59*, 1609–1613.

Campbell, J., & Leaver, J. (2003). Report from NTAC's national experts meeting on emerging new practices in organized peer support, March 17–18. Alexandria, VA. Retrieved from http://www.consumerstar.org/pubs/Emerging%20New%20Practices%20in%20Oraganized%20Peer%20Support.pdf.

Campbell, H. S., Phaneuf, M. R., & Deane, K. (2004). Cancer peer support programs—do they work? *Patient Education and Counseling, 55*, 3–15. doi:10.1016/j.pec.2003.10.001

Castillo, L. G., & Schwartz, S. J. (2013). College student mental health. *Journal of Clinical Psychology, 69*, 291–297. doi:10.1002/jclp.21972

Chartier, M. J., Walker, J. R., & Naimark, B. (2010). Separate and cumulative effects of adverse childhood experiences in predicting adult health and health care utilization. *Child Abuse & Neglect, 34*, 454–464. doi:10.1016/j.chiabu.2009.09.020

Cook, J. A., Copeland, M. E., Floyd, C. B., Jonikas, J. A., Hamilton, M. M., Razzano, L., … Boyd, S. (2012). A randomized controlled trial of effects of wellness recovery action planning on depression, anxiety, and recovery. *Psychiatric Services, 63*, 541–547. doi:10.1176/appi.ps.201100125

Daniels, A. S., Cate, R., Bergeson, S., Forquer, S., Niewenhous, G., & Epps, B. (2013). Best practices: Level-of-care criteria for peer support services: A best-practice guide. *Psychiatric Services (Washington, D.C.), 64*, 1190–1192. doi:10.1176/appi.ps.201300277

Davidson, L., Chinman, M., Sells, D., & Rowe, M. (2005). Peer support among adults with serious mental illness: A report from the field. *Schizophrenia Bulletin, 32*, 443–450. doi:10.1093/schbul/sbj043

Day, C., Michelson, D., Thomson, S., Penney, C., & Draper, L. (2012). Innovations in practice: Empowering parents, empowering communities: A pilot evaluation of a peer-led parenting programme: Empowering Parents, Empowering Communities programme. *Child and Adolescent Mental Health, 17*, 52–57. doi:10.1111/j.1475-3588.2011.00619.x

Eagan, K., Stolzenberg, E., B., Ramirez, J., J., Aragon, M., C., Suchard, M., R., & Hurtado, S. (2014). *The American freshman: National norms fall 2014*. Los Angeles: Higher Education Research Institute, UCLA.

Eisenberg, D., Golberstein, E., & Gollust, S. E. (2007). Help-seeking and access to mental health care in a university student population. *Medical Care, 45*, 594–601. doi:10.1097/MLR.0b013e31803bb4c1

Felitti, V., J., & Anda, R., F. (2010). The relationship of adverse childhood experiences to adult health, well-being, social function, and healthcare. In R. Lanius & E. Vermetten (Eds.), *The hidden epidemic: The impact of early life trauma on health and disease* (pp. 77–87). Cambridge, U.K.: Cambridge University Press.

Felitti, V. J., Anda, R. F., Nordenberg, D., Williamson, D. F., Spitz, A. M., Edwards, V., … Marks, J. S. (1998). Relationship of childhood abuse and household dysfunction to many of the leading causes of death in adults: The Adverse Childhood Experiences (ACE) Study. *American Journal of Preventive Medicine, 14*, 245–258. doi:10.1016/S0749-3797(98)00017-8

Felitti, V. J., & Williams, S. A. (1998). Long-term follow-up and analysis of more than 100 patients who each lost more than 100 pounds. *The Permanente Journal, 2*, 17–21.

Finkelhor, D., Shattuck, A., Turner, H., & Hamby, S. (2013). Improving the adverse childhood experiences study scale. *JAMA Pediatrics, 167*, 70. doi:10.1001/jamapediatrics.2013.420

Frese, F. J., Knight, E. L., & Saks, E. (2009). Recovery from schizophrenia: With views of psychiatrists, psychologists, and others diagnosed with this disorder. *Schizophrenia Bulletin, 35*, 370–380. doi:10.1093/schbul/sbn175

Gallagher, R. P. (2014). *National survey of college counseling centers (Monograph Series Number 9V)*. Alexandria, VA: The International Association of Counseling Services.

Goldstrom, I. D., Campbell, J., Rogers, J. A., Lambert, D. B., Blacklow, B., Henderson, M. J., & Manderscheid, R. W. (2006). National estimates for mental health mutual support groups, self-help organizations, and consumer-operated services. *Administration and Policy in Mental Health and Mental Health Services Research, 33*, 92–103. doi:10.1007/s10488-005-0019-x

Hardt, J., Vellaisamy, P., & Schoon, I. (2010). Sequelae of prospective versus retrospective reports of adverse childhood experiences. *Psychological Reports, 107*, 425–440. doi:10.2466/02.04.09.10.16.21.PR0.107.5.425-440

Herman, S., Archambeau, O. G., Deliramich, A. N., Kim, B. S. K., Chiu, P. H., & Frueh, B. C. (2011). Depressive symptoms and mental health treatment in an ethnoracially diverse college student sample. *Journal of American College Health, 59*, 715–720. doi:10.1080/07448481.2010.529625

Hunt, J., & Eisenberg, D. (2010). Mental health problems and help-seeking behavior among college students. *Journal of Adolescent Health, 46*, 3–10. doi:10.1016/j.jadohealth.2009.08.008

Kendall-Tackett, K. (2002). The health effects of childhood abuse: Four pathways by which abuse can influence health. *Child Abuse & Neglect, 26*, 715–729. doi:10.1016/S0145-2134(02)00343-5

Kessler, R. C., Berglund, P., Demler, O., Jin, R., Merikangas, K. R., & Walters, E. E. (2005). Lifetime prevalence and age-of-onset distributions of DSM-IV disorders in the National Comorbidity Survey Replication. *Archives of General Psychiatry, 62*, 593–602. doi:10.1001/archpsyc.62.6.593

Larkin, H., Shields, J. J., & Anda, R. F. (2012). The health and social consequences of Adverse Childhood Experiences (ACE) across the lifespan: An introduction to prevention and intervention in the community. *Journal of Prevention & Intervention in the Community, 40*, 263–270. doi:10.1080/10852352.2012.707439

Logan-Greene, P., Green, S., Nurius, P. S., & Longhi, D. (2014). Distinct contributions of adverse childhood experiences and resilience resources: A cohort analysis of adult physical and mental health. *Social Work in Health Care, 53*, 776–797. doi:10.1080/00981389.2014.944251

McGavock, L., & Spratt, T. (2014). Prevalence of adverse childhood experiences in a university population: Associations with use of social services. *British Journal of Social Work, 44*, 657–674. doi:10.1093/bjsw/bcs127

McLaughlin, K. A., Green, J. G., Gruber, M. J., Sampson, N. A., Zaslavsky, A. M., & Kessler, R. C. (2012). Childhood adversities and first onset of psychiatric disorders in a national sample of US adolescents. *Archives of General Psychiatry, 69*, 1151–1160. doi:10.1001/archgenpsychiatry.2011.2277

Mobile Digest of Education Statistics. (2013). Retrieved from http://nces.ed.gov/programs/digest/mobile/Enrollment_DGI_Enrollment_Rates_of_18_to_24_Year_Olds.aspx (Accessed May 27, 2016).

National Alliance on Mental Illness (n.d.). NAMI Peer-to-peer. Retrieved from http://www.nami.org/Find-Support/NAMI-Programs/NAMI-Peer-to-Peer (Accessed July 16, 2018).

Nemeroff, C. B., Heim, C. M., Thase, M. E., Klein, D. N., Rush, A. J., Schatzberg, A. F. … (2003). Differential responses to psychotherapy versus pharmacotherapy in patients with chronic forms of major depression and childhood trauma. *Proceedings of the National Academy of Sciences, 100*, 14293–14296. doi:10.1073/pnas.2336126100

R. CoreTeam. (2017). *R: A language and environment for statistical computing.* Vienna, Austria: R Foundation for Statistical Computing. Retrieved from https://www.R-project.org/

Read, J. P., Ouimette, P., White, J., Colder, C., & Farrow, S. (2011). Rates of DSM–IV–TR trauma exposure and posttraumatic stress disorder among newly matriculated college students. *Psychological Trauma: Theory, Research, Practice, and Policy, 3,* 148–156. doi:10.1037/a0021260

Smyth, J. M., Hockemeyer, J. R., Heron, K. E., Wonderlich, S. A., & Pennebaker, J. W. (2008). Prevalence, type, disclosure, and severity of adverse life events in college students. *Journal of American College Health, 57,* 69–76. doi:10.3200/JACH.57.1.69-76

Tang, T. S., Funnell, M. M., Gillard, M., Nwankwo, R., & Heisler, M. (2011). Training peers to provide ongoing diabetes self-management support (DSMS): Results from a pilot study. *Patient Education and Counseling, 85,* 160–168. doi:10.1016/j.pec.2010.12.013

Webel, A. R., Okonsky, J., Trompeta, J., & Holzemer, W. L. (2010). A systematic review of the effectiveness of peer-based interventions on health-related behaviors in adults. *American Journal of Public Health, 100,* 247. doi:10.2105/AJPH.2008.149419

World Health Organization. (1978). *International classification of diseases: [9th] ninth revision, basic tabulation list with alphabetic index.* Geneva, Switzerland: WHO. Retrieved from. http://www.who.int/iris/handle/10665/39473

Intergenerational Transmission of Depression during Adolescence: The Mediating Roles of Hostile Attribution Bias, Empathic Concern, and Social Self-concept

Xing Wei, Xi Li, Xiaoqin Teng, Jingyao Bai and Feifei Ren

ABSTRACT

Few studies have empirically examined the role of peer microsystem in the intergenerational transmission of depression, and more importantly, little is known about the mechanisms underlying this potential pathway of intergenerational transmission. The purpose of the current study was to examine the sequential mediation effects of adolescent hostile attribution bias, empathic concern, and social self-concept on the association between maternal depression and adolescent depression. An urban Chinese sample of 761 mother-child dyads was investigated when the adolescents were in secondary school ($M = 14.36$ years, range =12.33–16.92 years, 52.3% female). The results provided evidence of cross-generational continuity in depression during adolescence, and the hypothesized sequential mediation model was supported. The findings highlight the importance of peer-related factors during the intergenerational transmission of depression and have important implications for interpersonal interventions that aim to prevent depression during adolescence. The limitations of the study and suggestions for future research are briefly discussed.

Introduction

Depression is highly prevalent in puberty, and approximately 20–50% of adolescents experience pronounced depressive symptoms (Kessler et al., 2001). Adolescents with depression are more likely to have poor psychosocial functioning and academic achievement and a lower level of physical and mental health than other adolescents (Jaycox et al., 2009; López-López et al., 2021; Verboom et al., 2014). In addition, adolescents with depression are at an elevated risk of experiencing more chronic, severe, and impairing depressive symptoms in adulthood (Lieb et al., 2002). Many researchers have tried to identify the causes of depression, and some have concluded that the continuity of depression across generations may play a particularly important role (Goodman et al., 2011; Hammen et al., 2012). Goodman and Gotlib (1999) developed their Integrative Model and identified four major mediators of this intergenerational transmission: (a) the heritability of depression; (b) innate neuro regulatory dysfunction; (c) negative maternal affect, cognitions, and behaviors; and (d) a stressful family environment. Based on this theoretical explanation, prior studies have mainly focused on genetic and family factors when exploring how maternal depression affects offspring depression (Elmelid et al., 2015; Vaske et al., 2009). These findings shed light on the mechanisms through which maternal depression influences adolescent depression.

However, compared with the extensive research revealing the importance of family-relevant factors, little is known about the role of peer-relevant factors in the process of the intergenerational transmission of depression. In addition to parents, peers are one of the most crucial microsystems that affect children's depression, especially when these children enter puberty (Kochel et al., 2012; Platt et al., 2013). In explaining the mechanisms and factors of depression in individuals, the interpersonal risk model emphasizes that poor peer relations constitute a significant stressor that contributes to problematic outcomes, including depressive symptoms (Kochel et al., 2012; Patterson & Capaldi, 1990). Findings from several studies also support the proposition that poor peer relationships antecede the development of depressive symptoms in adolescents. For example, McDonald et al. (2010) found that the worse peer relationships are, the more likely an individual is to have psychological distress and become depressed and anxious during early adolescence. Fontaine et al. (2009) found that poor peer relationships have a negative influence on the development of psychological adjustment and problems such as depression. Thus, the role of peer relationships should not be overlooked in the intergenerational transmission of depression.

Hammen (1991) proposed an intergenerational interpersonal stress model of depression, which noted that youth's interpersonal functioning is a pathway for the intergenerational transmission of depression. The results of their empirical study further indicated that the negative effects of maternal depression on their offspring's depressive outcomes are largely mediated through the effect of maternal depression on youth's social competence with peers (Hammen et al., 2004). Similarly, studies have shown that adolescents of depressed mothers have poorer peer relationships and less adequate social skills than teens of non-depressed mothers (Goodman & Tully, 2006; Hammen & Brennan, 2003). Therefore, the current study focused on two important peer-relevant components concerning previous studies, one is peer-related emotional and cognitive psychosocial processes, and the other is peer relationships (Hay et al., 2004). Accordingly, the primary goal of the current study was to examine cross-generational continuity in depression during adolescence and to explore intergenerational transmission's mechanisms from the perspective of peer-related factors.

In the present study, we chose social self-concept as the index of adolescents' peer relationships. Social self-concept represents a person's self-perception of his or her social acceptance by others (Harter, 1996). Compared with objective measurements of peer relationships, such as friendship quality, popularity, and peer acceptance, social self-concept is more subjective. Given that depression is a self-perceived mood disorder, an individual's subjective perception of peer relationships might have a stronger relationship with depression. According to the competency-based model, negative events in a child's life, such as maternal depression, lead to maladaptive self-perceptions of the child's ability to function in the social domain (e.g. social self-concept), which may serve as a cognitive vulnerability factor for depression (Cole, 1990; Jacobs et al., 2008).

Class et al. (2012) used a quasi-experimental study and found that greater levels of maternal depressive symptoms were associated with lower levels of offspring's perceived self-competence scores. Spilt et al. (2014) found that children's social self-concept has negative effects on the development of internalizing problems. Thus, maternal depression may have an impact on adolescent depression by affecting adolescents' social self-concept.

When exploring the intergenerational transmission of depression from a peer-related perspective, another important question is how maternal depression affects perceived peer relationships and, subsequently, adolescent depression. Based on Roeser's (1996) Context-Process-Outcome Model, which stressed out the processes that link perceptions of the environment with developmental outcomes, the present study constructed the hypothetical model that maternal depression (family context) would first affect adolescents' cognitive and emotional factors (psychosocial mediating process) and then their social self-concept and depression (developmental outcomes). Previous studies have shown that the influence of maternal depression on adolescent peer relationships is often indirect and have identified adolescents' cognitive and emotional factors as mediators between maternal depression and youth social competence with peers. For example, studies have shown that emotional regulation, general self-concept, and executive functioning may play mediating roles in maternal depression and adolescent peer relationships (Deković & Meeus, 1997; Kam et al., 2011; Ladd & Pettit, 2002).

However, the cognitive and emotional factors explored in these studies are mostly on the individual level, which points to the individual self. While the factors on the interpersonal level, which point to the other person in the social interaction, may play a more important role in the formation of one's socialization and social self-concept (Khan et al., 2016; Trigueros et al., 2020). Wang and Dix's research (2015) shows that mothers with depressive symptoms place children at risk of developing maladaptive social cognition, and it predicts children's low social competence 4 years later in first grade. Scherer et al. (2019) found that maternal depressive symptoms are associated with children's poorer social-emotional development. Furthermore, adolescents' higher level of social-emotional factors has been shown to predict positive peer relationships (DeLay et al., 2016). Therefore, the cognitive and emotional factors of peer interactions could be potential mediators between maternal depression and adolescents' peer relationships. Moreover, because most studies to date have examined cognitive and emotional factors in isolation from one another, the simultaneous effect of interpersonal-related cognitive and emotional factors on adolescent social self-concept, as well as on adolescent depression, could be tested in the present study.

Regarding the cognitive factors of peer interactions, hostile attribution bias is one that is closely related to peer relationships (Dodge et al., 2003). Hostile attribution bias refers to the tendency to interpret ambiguous stimuli in terms of hostility and aggression (Krahé & Möller, 2004). Research reveals that depressed mothers are less positively engaged with their children and demonstrate a high level of rejection and psychological control (Aunola et al., 2015; Henry et al., 2020; Rohrer et al., 2011). The child's negative perception of such parent-child interactions is likely to cause more negative relational schemas and scripts, which in turn lead to biased hostile social cognitions toward their peers (Gomez et al., 2001). Using data from the NICHD Study of Early Child Care, Wang and Dix (2015) found that maladaptive social cognition (with hostile attribution bias as one of the three cognition components) mediated relations between mothers' early depressive symptoms and children's low first-grade social competence. Based on the previous findings, we hypothesized a cognitive pathway in which maternal depression affects adolescent social self-concept indirectly through its effect on hostile attribution bias.

Concerning the emotional factors of peer interactions, empathic concern is considered to be essentially linked to peer relationships (Boele et al., 2019). Empathic concern is the tendency to feel compassion, sympathy, and concern when encountering others (Davis, 1983). It originates and forms in the family context (Koestner et al., 1990; Zahn-Waxler & Radke-Yarrow, 1990) and is an important socio-emotional factor related to adolescent social relationships (George-Levi et al., 2021; Guild et al., 2017). Nevertheless, mixed findings have been reported in previous investigations that have explored how maternal depression affects adolescents' peer relationships through empathic concern. For example, some studies suggest that young children of depressed mothers who overemphasize their parents' distressed and unhappy feelings may themselves experience too much distress and confuse boundaries between themselves and significant others. Such conditions would be expected to interfere with social interaction patterns with peers (Zahn-Waxler & Radke-Yarrow, 1990). Thus, maternal depression may compromise adolescents' social competence through the child's higher level of empathic responses to their mother's distress. Recent empirical studies have reported that maternal depression, especially chronic maternal depression, is negatively related to children's social-emotional adjustment because the family environment hosted by depressed mothers undermines the development of adolescent empathic concern (Tully & Donohue, 2017). Children's poor empathic concern commonly predicts subsequent worse peer relations in adolescence (Ladd et al., 1999). The reason for these inconsistent findings might be that previous studies mainly focused on the child's perception of the mother's pain, while little attention has been given to how mothers' depression affects children's response to other people's pain, especially that of peers (Zahn-Waxler et al., 1990; Zahn-Waxler & Kochanska, 1988; Zahn-Waxler & Radke-Yarrow, 1990). Thus, in the present study, we speculated that empathic concern may mediate associations between maternal depression and children's social self-concept. However, we did not have a specific hypothesis concerning the directions of the mediating pathways because prior results are mixed.

Finally, most research in this area was conducted in Western settings, and little is known about this issue in Chinese societies. Given the unique Chinese cultural values in the interpersonal context, great importance is placed on the harmony of interpersonal relationships (Leung et al., 2011). As a result, poor interpersonal relationships may lead to more maladaptive problems, especially in adolescents. Specifically, when adolescents have problems with peer relationships, they may have more difficulty adjusting to school life, lack peers support when encountering difficulties, and be more likely to experience depression (Hawker & Boulton, 2000; Nansel et al., 2001). In addition, Chinese adolescents are currently more likely to have problems in peer relationships because of their focus on academic performance since secondary school, which stems from increasing academic pressure and insufficient peer interaction. Therefore, it is meaningful to examine the intergenerational transmission of depression from a peer perspective in the Chinese cultural context.

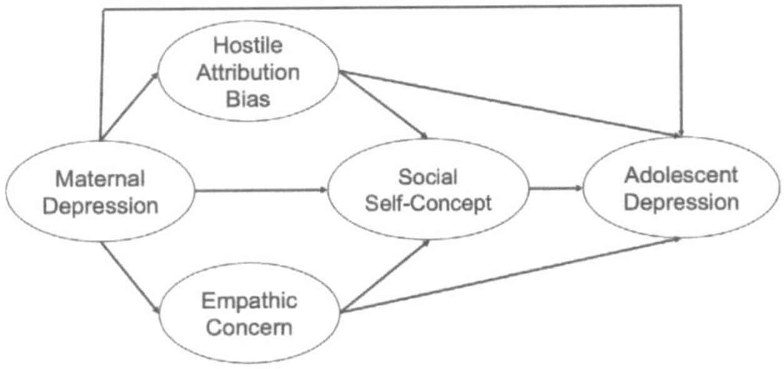

Figure 1. The hypothesized sequential mediation model.

In summary, the current study aimed to examine the intergenerational transmission of depression from a peer perspective and whether the intergenerational transmission of depression is sequentially mediated by adolescents' hostile attribution bias, empathic concern, and social self-concept. Specifically, we hypothesized that maternal depression affects adolescents' hostile attribution bias and empathic concern toward peers, which in turn affects adolescents' social self-concept and, ultimately, adolescents' depression. A detailed hypothetical model of the three-path mediating effects of empathic concern, hostile attribution bias, and social self-concept on relationships in the intergenerational transmission of depression is presented in Figure 1.

Methods

Participants

Data were collected from seventh-, eighth- and ninth-grade students at two public middle schools in Shandong Province in eastern China. A total of 761 students participated in this study. All the participants lived in urban areas in the cities of Qingdao and Zibo. Of the 761 participants who were recruited, 34 did not report their age. The mean age was 14.36 years (SD =.94), with 11.6% 12-year-olds ($n=84$), 35.3% 13-year-olds ($n=257$), 34.9% 14-year-olds ($n=254$), 17.6% 15-year-olds ($n=128$), and 0.6% 16-year-olds ($n=4$). Among the sample, 398 were girls (52.30%) and 362 were boys. Regarding the educational level of the mothers, 23.76% of mothers had an educational level ranging from college to university graduate or higher, and the remainder had completed senior high school education or less. The monthly combined family income of the sample was as follows: 38.15% of the families had income above ¥7000, 27.37% of the families had income between ¥5000 and ¥7000, and the remainder had income below ¥5000. In terms of these demographic variables, this sample was similar to the urban population in East China (The National Bureau of Statistics of the People's Republic of China, 2018), suggesting that it was representative of at least the urban population in China.

Procedure

The study was approved by the local ethics committee. Informed assent (children) and consent (mothers and school principals) were obtained before data collection. After obtaining parental informed consent, a packet containing the mother's questionnaires was sent home with the participating adolescents. The mothers were instructed by the teachers within a specified time to complete the questionnaires through the online WeChat group at home and return them to school in sealed envelopes. In the attached instructions, mothers were made aware of the voluntary and confidential nature of this research. In addition, questionnaires were administered to groups of adolescents by two trained research assistants in separate classrooms, and the adolescents independently completed the questionnaires during classroom hours or immediately after school.

Measures

Maternal Depression

Maternal depression was assessed by depression subscale of the Personal Disturbance Scale (sAD), a brief 14-item self-report measure of depression and anxiety derived from the Delusions–Symptoms States Inventory (DSSI; Bedford & Foulds, 1978). Studies have shown that the sAD possess adequate internal consistencies (Bedford & Deary, 1999; Christensen et al., 1999). The correlations among sAD and other depression scales such as Hospital Anxiety and Depression Scale (HADS; Zigmond & Snaith, 1983) and the Depression sub-scales of Depression Anxiety Stress Scales (DASS; Lovibond & Lovibond, 1995) were all highly significant, supporting the validatory evidence for sAD (Henry et al., 2002). Data of both anxiety subscale and depression subscale was collected with the current sample but only data of depression subscale was used to assess maternal depression. The depression subscale contains 7 items such as "In the recent past, I have felt that there is little hope for the future" and "In the recent past, I feel panic with no reason". The average score for all items represents the frequency of maternal depressive symptoms or depressive status and the degree of personality disorder (0 = False, 1 = Occasionally, 2 = Frequently, 3 = Always). Higher scores indicate more severe depressive symptoms. To adapt the questionnaire to Chinese, a translation/back-translation process was carried out by bilingual translators and experts in the field. The resulting questionnaire was revised by another two psychological experts. Finally, the resulting version was revised once again by the research group and an additional translator to ensure that conceptual equivalence had been maintained throughout all phases of the process. Slight modifications were made to ensure content validity. Cronbach's alpha for this questionnaire was .839 in this study.

Hostile Attribution Bias

Adolescents' hostile attribution bias toward their peers was measured using a hostile attribution type questionnaire developed by Krahé and Möller (2004). The questionnaire used 4 scenarios to measure adolescents' tendency to interpret ambiguous interactions in a hostile fashion. These scenarios described some form of harm to the target classmate, but it is not obvious whether this harm was intentional. Two scenarios described situations in which the target classmate suffered physical harm or damage to his or her property (e.g. "A student runs over in a hurry and knocks your books and notebooks to the floor"), and two scenarios described a relational problem (e.g. "You hear two of your classmates mention your name, and as you walk toward them, they suddenly stop talking"). Following the scenario, participants were asked to provide ratings on three dimensions: perceived hostile intent, anger, and wish to retaliate. The questionnaire was scored with 3 points ranging from 0 to 2 for "not at all" to "very much". Higher scores indicate a higher level of hostile attribution bias. Cronbach's alpha for this questionnaire was .843 in this study.

Empathic Concern

Empathic concern was assessed with the empathic concern subscale of Interpersonal Reactivity Index (IRI, Davis's,1980), which is a self-reported questionnaire consisting of four 7-item subscales, including Fantasy (FS), Perspective Taking (PT), Empathetic Concern (EC), and Personal Distress (PD). In the current study, only the scores of EC subscale and PT subscale were collected. Specifically, perspective taking is a kind of cognitive empathy refers to the understanding of another person's feelings, while empathic concern is a kind of affective empathy means feeling sorrow or concern for the observed other (Boele et al., 2019). Since the present study is concerned with the emotional ability of adolescents, only the score of EC subscale was used in the data analysis. Evidence for validity is extensive for EC subscale (Murphy et al., 2020), and there are also findings supporting the validity of the EC subscale in a Chinese sample (Siu & Shek, 2005). To limit empathic concern to the peer context in the current study, the description of the items were briefly modified so that middle school students could report how they would emotionally react to the negative experiences of their peers (e.g. "I often care about those students who are not as lucky as me"). All items were rated on a scale ranging from 1 ("does not describe me well") to 5 ("describes me very well"), with higher scores indicating a higher level of empathic concern. Cronbach's alpha for the EC scale was .652 in this study.

Social Self-Concept

Social self-concept was measured using the social perceived competence subscale from the Self-Perception Profile for Children (Harter, 1985),which contains 6 subscales including scholastic competence, social perceived competence, athletic competence, physical appearance, behavioral conduct and global self-worth. Evidence for construct validity and adequate reliability was found for each subscale (Harter, 2012). The SPPC is a commonly used measure of self-concept in children (Cheong & Johnston, 2013). Of particular interest in this study were children's perceptions of their own competence in the social domain. Accordingly, although the measure was administered in its entirety, only score of social perceived competence was considered in data analyses.

The social perceived competence subscale contains 6 items. For each item, adolescents were given a description of two people, one who was doing well in the relevant domain and another who was not (e.g. "I am popular in my class" vs. "I am not popular in my class"). Participants were then asked which of the two people they most resembled and whether the description was "really true for me" or "sort of true for me". Each item was then rated from 1 to 4, with higher scores indicating more positive self-perception. Cronbach's alpha for this subscale was .874 in this study.

Adolescent Depression

Adolescent depression was measured using the mother-reported version of the Child Behavior Checklist (CBCL; Achenbach & Edelbrock, 1985). It has been proved that the Child Behavior Checklist is a widely used questionnaire to assess behavioral and emotional problems (Achenbach, 2019). The Child Behavior Checklist contains 8 subscales including anxious/depressed, withdrawn/depressed, somatic complaints, social problems, thought problems, attention problems, rule-breaking behavior, and aggressive behavior. Studies have shown that the scale has good reliability and validity and is suitable for use in Chinese cultural contexts (Mazefsky et al., 2011; Xing et al., 2011). Based on the ASEBA DSM-oriented scales for DSM-5 criteria (Achenbach, 2013), the Depressive Problems Scale consists of 13 items, such as "There is very little he/she enjoys", "Cries a lot", "Feels worthless or inferior". The items were rated on a scale ranging from 0 ("not true") to 2 ("very true or often true"). Higher scores reflect more severe depressive problems. Cronbach's alpha for it was .75 in this study.

Statistical Analyses

Preliminarily, multivariate multiple regression analysis was performed to examine whether there were any statistically significant associations between demographic characteristics (including adolescent age, gender, only child, and socioeconomic status) and adolescent depression to decide whether covariates were needed. Then, a Pearson correlation coefficient was computed to examine the associations between variables.

We conducted structural equation modeling (SEM) analysis using the Mplus 7 statistical software package to test our sequential mediation model (Muthén & Muthén, 1998–2015). Full information maximum likelihood (FIML) estimation was used to handle missing data. Before examining the hypothesized model, the structural validity of each latent factor was tested with confirmatory factor analysis (CFA). However, in the final structural model, an item parceling process was utilized for several latent constructs to reduce the number of indicators and increase reliability (Little et al., 2002; Yang et al., 2010). By using a factorial algorithm (Rogers & Schmitt, 2004), factor analysis was first conducted to determine how many equivalent parts (parcels) each latent variable could be split into. Then, items with similar loadings in the scale were parceled into the same dimension. All parcels presented significant loadings in the calculated structural equation model. The advantages of creating parcels of related items is that true error variance and item-specific variance are minimized, whereas true score variance is increased (Little et al., 2002). Parcels also typically produce more stable solutions than do the individual scale items.

The overall model fit was assessed using the following fit indices and recommended cutoff values: (1) the chi-square statistic and normed chi-square (χ^2/df), (2) the comparative fit index (CFI), and (3) the root mean square error of approximation (RMSEA). The model fit is considered good when the χ^2/df ratio is less than 3, the CFI is above .95 and the RMSEA is below .05 (Hu & Bentler, 1999). The significance of mediation effects was tested using product-of-coefficients tests for two-path (single mediator) and three-path (two mediators in series) mediated effects (Taylor et al., 2008). Bootstrapped confidence intervals (CIs) were used to determine the significance of the mediated effects.

Table 1. Means, Standard Deviations, and Bivariate Correlations between Study Variables.

	M	*SD*	1	2	3	4	5
1. Maternal depression	0.12	0.28	—				
2. Empathic concern	2.67	0.64	-.10**	—			
3. Hostile attribution bias	0.56	0.38	.10**	-.14**	—		
4. Social self-concept	2.30	0.49	-.03	.23**	-.17**	—	
5. Adolescent depression	0.18	0.22	.27**	.07*	.09*	-.16**	—

*Correlation is significant at the .05 level (2-tailed).
**Correlation is significant at the .01 level (2-tailed).

Results

Descriptive Statistics

Preliminary analyses indicated no significant associations between demographic characteristics (i.e. adolescent age, gender, only child, and socioeconomic status) and adolescent depression; thus, no covariates were included in the following analysis. Table 1 presents the means, standard deviations, and zero-order correlations of all study variables. The mean score of maternal depression in the current study is a little lower than previous studies in western samples (ranging from 0.16 ~ 0.31, Bedford & Deary, 1997; Henry et al., 2002), but is similar to previous study in a Chinese sample ($M = 0.10$, Yang et al., 2017). The mean score of hostile attribution bias was a little lower than previous studies in western samples($M = 0.81$; Möller & Krahé, 2009). Compared with previous studies using Chinese samples, the mean score of empathic concern ($M = 2.70$; Zhang et al., 2021), social self-concept($M = 2.85$; Zhang et al., 2014) and adolescent depression($M = 0.28$; Yang et al., 2017) are all slightly lower in the current study. The results of bivariate correlation analysis showed that adolescent depression was significantly and positively correlated with maternal depression and hostile attribution bias and significantly and negatively correlated with social self-concept but not correlated with empathic concern. Social self-concept was significantly and negatively correlated with hostile attribution bias but positively correlated with empathic concern.

Sequential Mediation Model

The measurement model we used in this study consisted of 5 latent constructs (maternal depression, empathic concern, hostile attribution bias, social self-concept, and adolescent depression) and 13 observed indicators. All the factor loadings of the indicators of the latent variables were significant, indicating that all the latent factors were well represented by their respective indicators. The hypothesized model (see Figure 2) provided a good fit to the data (χ^2 = 140.07, df = 45, χ^2/df = 3.1; RMSEA =.053, 90% CI [.043, .063]; CFI =.97; Tucker–Lewis index (TLI) =.95).

As depicted in Figure 2, the model showed that maternal depression was significantly and positively associated with adolescent depression (β =.43, p <.001). Maternal depression was associated with both adolescent empathic concern and hostile attribution bias (empathic concern: β = −.15, p<.05; hostile attribution bias: β =.13, p<.001), whereas maternal depression was not significantly related to adolescent social self-concept (β =.04, p >.05). Empathic concern was significantly and positively related to adolescent

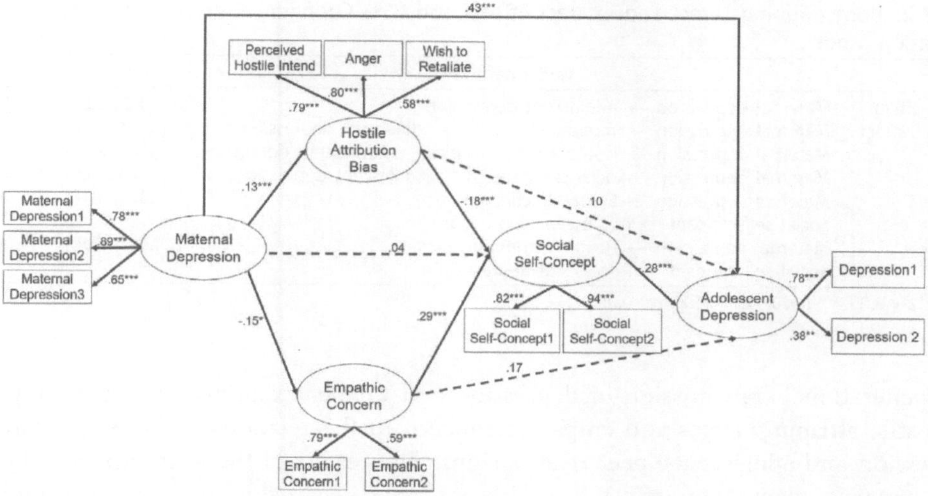

Figure 2. Final model concerning the sequential mediation effects of hostile attribution bias, empathic concern, and social self-concept on the relationships between maternal depression and adolescent depression.
Note. Solid arrows represent statistically significant pathways; dotted arrows represent nonsignificant pathways. The path coefficients are standardized.
*p <.05, **p <.01, ***p <.001.

social self-concept (β =.29, p <.001), whereas empathic concern was not significantly associated with an increase in adolescent depression (β =.17, p >.05). Hostile attribution bias was significantly and positively related to adolescent social self-concept (β = −.18, p <.001) but was not significantly related to an increase in adolescent depression (β =.10, p >.05). Social self-concept was significantly and positively associated with adolescent depression (β = −.28, p <.001).

Mediation analyses revealed that the two-path mediation effect of hostile attribution bias was not significant in the relationship between maternal depression and adolescent depression (β =.005, SE =.004, p =.19, 95% CI: [.000, .015]), and that of empathic concern was also not significant (β = −.010, SE =.008, p =.202, 95% CI: [-.034, −.001]). The other two-path mediation effect, involving maternal depression → social self-concept → adolescent depression, was not significant (β = −.004, SE =.008, p =.576, 95% CI: [-.023, .009]). The three-path mediation effect involving maternal depression → hostile attribution bias → social self-concept → adolescent depression was marginally significant (β =.004, SE =.001, p =.056, 95% CI: [.001, .010]). Another three-path mediation effect involving maternal depression → empathic concern → social self-concept → adolescent depression was significant (β =.007, SE =.003, p =.045, 95% CI: [.001, .018]) (Table 2).

Discussion

Little research has examined the mechanisms of the intergenerational transmission of depression from a peer-related perspective. This study contributed to the existing literature by examining the perceived peer relationship as the mechanism of

Table 2. Bootstrapping Direct and Indirect Effects and 95% Confidence Intervals (CIs) for the Final Mediation Model.

	Model pathways	95% CI	β
Direct effect	Maternal depression → Adolescent depression	[.063, .283]	.170**
Indirect effect	Maternal depression →Empathic concern → Adolescent depression	[-.034, .-001]	-.010
	Maternal depression →Hostile attribution bias → Adolescent depression	[.000, .015]	.005
	Maternal depression →Social self-concept → Adolescent depression	[-.023, .009]	-.004
	Maternal depression → Empathic concern → Social self-concept → Adolescent depression	[.001, .018]	.007*
	Maternal depression → Hostile attribution bias→ Social self-concept → Adolescent depression	[.001, .010]	.004†

Note. *$p < 0.05$. ** $p < 0.01$. † $0.10 > p > 0.05$.

intergenerational transmission of depression and further examined the mediating role of hostile attribution bias and empathic concern in the relationship between maternal depression and adolescents' peer relationships. The results of the current study showed that maternal depression affected adolescents' hostile attribution bias and empathic concern and was related to a lower level of social self-concept of adolescents, further adversely affecting adolescent depression. The findings of the current study support the interpersonal risk model and suggest that it is of great research significance to explore the mechanism of the intergenerational transmission of depression from a peer-related perspective. The above results are discussed in detail below.

Consistent with our hypothesis, in addition to confirming that maternal depression has a direct influence on adolescent depression (Goodman et al., 2011), we found a dual-pathway sequential mediation model with peer-related variables as mediators. For the first mediating pathway, we found that maternal depression, through adolescent hostile attribution bias and then social self-concept, affects adolescent depression. This result is in line with previous findings (Wang & Dix, 2015). The interaction of depressed mothers with their children in daily life is mostly negative (Kochanska, 2002; Lovejoy et al., 2000), and children in adolescence are more sensitive to parents' negative parenting behaviors (Mennen et al., 2018). Depressed mothers' low response and less attention to adolescents facilitate adolescents' development of negative cognition (Goodman et al., 2020), making adolescents more sensitive and hostile to others' reactions. According to social information processing theory, adolescents who lack or are biased in processing social information are likely to encounter difficulties in interacting with their peers and are evaluated negatively by their peers. This changes adolescents' cognition in relation to interpersonal communication and makes adolescents pay more attention to negative interactions and respond negatively to their peers. Failure to establish good peer relationships can further cause depression in adolescents (Spilt et al., 2014). Furthermore, while most previous studies have examined the indirect effect of a stressful family environment on the interaction between maternal depression and adolescent peer-related factors (Goodman et al., 2011; Hammen et al., 2004), the results of this study indicate that it is equally important to pay attention to the direct effect of maternal depression on peer-related factors.

The other sequential mediating pathway is maternal depression through adolescent empathic concern and then adolescent social self-concept to affect adolescent depression. This finding may suggest that adolescents of depressed mothers are likely to experience fewer feelings of sympathy and compassion for their peers, which is related to a lower level of social self-concept and a high level of adolescent depression. However, this result stands in contrast to that of the report by Zahn-Waxler et al. (1990), which showed that maternal depression increased adolescent empathic concern. One possible explanation for this inconsistency might be that previous studies on maternal depression affecting children's empathy or empathic concerns mainly focused on adolescents' perception of their mothers' pain (Zahn-Waxler et al., 1990; Zahn-Waxler & Kochanska, 1988; Zahn-Waxler & Radke-Yarrow, 1990), while empathic concern in the present study measured the degree of empathic concern of adolescents toward their peers. The inconsistent results may suggest that when mothers are depressed, adolescents pay too much attention to the mother's pain and ignore the concerns of their peers; therefore, maternal depression could affect adolescent depression through empathic concern toward both mothers and peers, but in different directions. Overall, the findings of this study support the crucial importance of both adolescent hostile attribution bias and empathic concern in the intergenerational transmission of depression.

Notably, we also found several non-significant direct effects in the present study. Our results showed that the influence of maternal depression on social self-concept was fully mediated by hostile attribution bias and empathic concern, and the influence of hostile attribution bias and empathic concern on adolescent depression was also fully mediated by social self-concept. These findings are consistent with those of prior empirical studies showing that the links between maternal or child depression and peer-related factors are indirect (Hammen et al., 2004; Laursen & Hartl, 2013; Witvliet et al.,2010). For example, Hammen et al. (2004) found that the link between maternal and child depression was entirely mediated by interpersonal and contextual factors. These results again highlight the important role of adolescents' cognitive and emotional factors in peer interactions and peer relationships in the intergenerational transmission of depression, especially for adolescents in Chinese culture. Because Chinese culture emphasizes collectivist values and cooperation in interpersonal relationships, the influence of peer relationships on depression may be more important for Chinese adolescents. However, given the lack of comparison groups from Western societies, further cross-cultural research is needed to explore cultural differences in the association between peer relationships and adolescent depression. Overall, maternal depression have a severe negative influence on adolescents' cognitive and emotional factors, which is related to fragile peer relationships and a higher level of depressive symptoms in adolescents. These findings reveal the complex mechanism of the intergenerational transmission of depression and further emphasize the necessity of using a multiple sequential mediation model to examine this problem.

Implications, Limitations and Future Directions

The findings of the present study are supported by several strengths. First, given that adolescence is a period of immense developmental change, this study highlights the intergenerational transmission of depression during adolescence. Second, this study explored the mechanism of intergenerational transmission of depression from the peer perspective, while most previous studies have focused on the protective and interventional role of the family. Finally, the role of peer-related cognitive and emotional factors in the intergenerational transmission of depression was clarified in the present study, providing an empirical basis for intervention practice in adolescent depression. For example, interventions can be used to help adolescents develop positive attribution styles or better emotional socialization or help them form better peer relationships to mitigate the negative effects of maternal depression.

Despite these advantages, several limitations also remain. First, the study adopted a cross-sectional research design. Although the existing theory and empirical evidence provided a solid foundation for this study, it was difficult to infer the causal relationship between the variables. Given the cross-sectional research design, the reciprocal relation between adolescents' empathic concern, hostile attribution bias and social self-concept could not be tested in the current study. Thus, alternative relations of the variables in the present study are possible. Adolescents with better self-concept may have greater empathic abilities and less hostile toward others (Castro-Sánchez et al., 2019). Longitudinal studies are required to provide more information on the cause-effect among variables in the future. Investigation and verification through the combination of experiments and follow-up studies are required to reveal the mechanism of action between the variables. Second, other microsystems were not included in this study while exploring peer factors. As a result, the joint effect and the interactions among different microsystems remain unclear. Future research could incorporate multiple microsystems, such as school and community systems, to examine the interaction of multiple systems. Finally, the current sample consisted mainly of parents of adolescents. It is not clear whether our findings can be generalized to parents of younger or older children. Additionally, it is worth noting that our sample is representative of Chinese urban families; thus, it remains to be seen whether these findings can be extended to families with various backgrounds.

Funding

This work was supported by Social Science Planning Project of Shandong Province (19DJY02, 20DJYJ04).

References

Achenbach, T. M. (2013). *DSM guide for the ASEBA*. University of Vermont, Research Center for Children, Youth, & Families.

Achenbach, T. M. (2019, March 12). *Aseba overview*. ASEBA. Retrieved July 23, 2022, from https://aseba.org/aseba-overview/

Achenbach, T. M., & Edelbrock, C. S. (1985). *Manual for the child behavior checklist and revised child behavior profile*. University Associates in Psychiatry.

Aunola, K., Ruusunen, A. K., Viljaranta, J., & Nurmi, J. E. (2015). Parental affection and psychological control as mediators between parents' depressive symptoms and child distress. *Journal of Family Issues*, *36*(8), 1022–1042. https://doi.org/10.1177/0192513X13494825

Bedford, A., & Deary, I. J. (1997). The Personal Disturbance Scale (DSSI/sAD): Development, use and structure. *Personality and Individual Differences*, *22*(4), 493–510. https://doi.org/10.1016/S0191-8869(96)00242-5

Bedford, A., & Deary, I. J. (1999). The Delusions-Symptoms-States Inventory (DSSI): Construction, applications and structural analyses. *Personality and Individual Differences*, *26*(3), 397–424. https://doi.org/10.1016/S0191-8869(98)00118-4

Bedford, A., & Foulds, G. (1978). *Delusions–symptoms–states inventory state of anxiety and depression*. NFER-Nelson.

Boele, S., Van der Graaff, J., de Wied, M., Van der Valk, I. E., Crocetti, E., & Branje, S. (2019). Linking parent–child and peer relationship quality to empathy in adolescence: A multilevel meta-analysis. *Journal of Youth and Adolescence*, *48*(6), 1033–1055. https://doi.org/10.1007/s10964-019-00993-5

Castro-Sánchez, M., Zurita-Ortega, F., Ruiz, G. R., & Chacón-Cuberos, R. (2019). Explanatory model of violent behaviours, self-concept and empathy in schoolchildren. Structural equations analysis. *Plos One*, *14*(8), e0217899. https://doi.org/10.1371/journal.pone.0217899

Cheong, S. K., & Johnston, L. M. (2013). Systematic review of self-concept measures for primary school aged children with cerebral palsy. *Research in Developmental Disabilities*, *34*(10), 3566–3575. https://doi.org/10.1016/j.ridd.2013.07.023

Christensen, H., Jorm, A. F., Mackinnon, A. J., Korten, A. E., Jacomb, P. A., Henderson, A. S., & Rodgers, B. (1999). Age differences in depression and anxiety symptoms: A structural equation modelling analysis of data from a general population sample. *Psychological Medicine*, *29*(2), 325–339. https://doi.org/10.1017/s0033291798008150

Class, Q. A., D'Onofrio, B. M., Singh, A. L., Ganiban, J. M., Spotts, E. L., Lichtenstein, P., Reiss, D., & Neiderhiser, J. M. (2012). Current parental depression and offspring perceived self-competence: A quasi-experimental examination. *Behavior Genetics*, *42*(5), 787–797. https://doi.org/10.1007/s10519-012-9550-1

Cole, D. A. (1990). Relation of social and academic competence to depressive symptoms in childhood. *Journal of Abnormal Psychology*, *99*(4), 422–429. https://doi.org/10.1037/0021-843X.99.4.422

Davis, M. H. (1980). A multidimensional approach to individual differences in empathy. *JSAS Catalog of Selected Documents in Psychology*, *10*, 85.

Davis, M. H. (1983). Empathic concern and the muscular dystrophy telethon: Empathy as a multidimensional construct. *Personality and Social Psychology Bulletin*, *9*(2), 223–229. https://doi.org/10.1177/0146167283092005

Deković, M., & Meeus, W. (1997). Peer relations in adolescence: Effects of parenting and adolescents' self-concept. *Journal of Adolescence*, *20*(2), 163–176. https://doi.org/10.1006/jado.1996.0074

DeLay, D., Zhang, L., Hanish, L. D., Miller, C. F., Fabes, R. A., Martin, C. L., Kochel, K. P., & Updegraff, K. A. (2016). Peer influence on academic performance: A Social network analysis of social-emotional intervention effects. *Prevention Science: The Official Journal of the Society for Prevention Research*, *17*(8), 903–913. https://doi.org/10.1007/s11121-016-0678-8

Dodge, K. A., Lansford, J. E., Burks, V. S., Bates, J. E., Pettit, G. S., Fontaine, R., & Price, J. M. (2003). Peer rejection and social information-processing factors in the development of aggressive behavior problems in children. *Child Development, 74*(2), 374–393. https://doi.org/10.1111/1467-8624.7402004

Elmelid, A., Stickley, A., Lindblad, F., Schwab-Stone, M., Henrich, C. C., & Ruchkin, V. (2015). Depressive symptoms, anxiety and academic motivation in youth: Do schools and families make a difference? *Journal of Adolescence, 45*, 174–182. https://doi.org/10.1016/j.adolescence.2015.08.003

Fontaine, R. G., Yang, C., Burks, V. S., Dodge, K. A., Price, J. M., Pettit, G. S., & Bates, J. E. (2009). Loneliness as a partial mediator of the relation between low social preference in childhood and anxious/depressed symptoms in adolescence. *Development and Psychopathology, 21*(2), 479–491. https://doi.org/10.1017/S0954579409000261

George-Levi, S., Laslo-Roth, R., & Schmidt-Barad, T. (2021). Feeling you, when you feel me: Attachment, empathic concern, and interpersonal emotion regulation. *The Journal of Social Psychology*. Advance online publication. https://doi.org/10.1080/00224545.2021.1940075

Gomez, R., Gomez, A., Demello, L., & Tallent, R. (2001). Perceived maternal control and support: Effects on hostile biased social information processing and aggression among clinic-referred children with high aggression. *Journal of Child Psychology and Psychiatry, 42*(4), 513–522. https://doi.org/10.1111/1469-7610.00745

Goodman, S. H., & Gotlib, I. H. (1999). Risk for psychopathology in the children of depressed mothers: A developmental model for understanding mechanisms of transmission. *Psychological Review, 106*(3), 458–490.

Goodman, S. H., & Tully, E. (2006). Depression in Women Who Are Mothers: An Integrative Model of Risk for the Development of Psychopathology in Their Sons and Daughters. In C. L. M. Keyes & S. H. Goodman (Eds.), *Women and depression: A handbook for the social, behavioral, and biomedical sciences* (pp. 241–280). Cambridge University Press. https://doi.org/10.1017/CBO9780511841262.013

Goodman, S. H., Rouse, M. H., Connell, A. M., Broth, M. R., Hall, C. M., & Heyward, D. (2011). Maternal depression and child psychopathology: A meta-analytic review. *Clinical Child and Family Psychology Review, 14*(1), 1–27.

Goodman, S. H., Simon, H. F., Shamblaw, A. L., & Kim, C. Y. (2020). Parenting as a mediator of associations between depression in mothers and children's functioning: A systematic review and meta-analysis. *Clinical Child and Family Psychology Review, 23*(4), 427–460. https://doi.org/10.1007/s10567-020-00322-4

Guild, D. J., Toth, S. L., Handley, E. D., Rogosch, F. A., & Cicchetti, D. (2017). Attachment security mediates the longitudinal association between child-parent psychotherapy and peer relations for toddlers of depressed mothers. *Development and Psychopathology, 29*(2), 587–600. https://doi.org/10.1017/S0954579417000207

Hammen, C. (1991). Generation of stress in the course of unipolar depression. *Journal of Abnormal Psychology, 100*(4), 555–561. https://doi.org/10.1037//0021-843X.100.4.555

Hammen, C., & Brennan, P. A. (2003). Severity, chronicity, and timing of maternal depression and risk for adolescent offspring diagnoses in a community sample. *Archives of General Psychiatry, 60*(3), 253–258. https://doi.org/10.1001/archpsyc.60.3.253

Hammen, C., Hazel, N. A., Brennan, P. A., & Najman, J. (2012). Intergenerational transmission and continuity of stress and depression: Depressed women and their offspring in 20 years of follow-up. *Psychological Medicine, 42*(5), 931–942. https://doi.org/10.1017/s0033291711001978

Hammen, C., Shih, J. H., & Brennan, P. A. (2004). Intergenerational transmission of depression: Test of an interpersonal stress model in a community sample. *Journal of Consulting and Clinical Psychology, 72*(3), 511–522. https://doi.org/10.1037/0022-006X.72.3.511

Harter, S. (1985). *Manual for self-perception profile for children*. University of Denver.

Harter, S. (1996). Historical roots of contemporary issues involving self-concept. In B. A. Bracken (Ed.), *Handbook of self-concept: Developmental, social, and clinical considerations* (pp. 1–37). John Wiley & Sons.

Harter, S. (2012). *Self-perception profile for children: Manual and questionnaires*. Univeristy of Denver, Department of Psychology.

Hawker, D. S., & Boulton, M. J. (2000). Twenty years' research on peer victimization and psychosocial maladjustment: A meta-analytic review of cross-sectional studies. *Journal of Child Psychology and Psychiatry, and Allied Disciplines*, *41*(4), 441–455.

Hay, D. F., Payne, A., & Chadwick, A. (2004). Peer relations in childhood. *Journal of Child Psychology and Psychiatry, and Allied Disciplines*, *45*(1), 84–108. https://doi.org/10.1046/j.0021-9630.2003.00308.x

Henry, J. D., Crawford, J. R., Bedford, A., Crombie, C. M., & Taylor, E. P. (2002). The personal disturbance scale (sAD): Normative data and latent structure in a large non-clinical sample. *Personality and Individual Differences*, *33*(8), 1343–1360. https://doi.org/10.1016/S0191-8869(02)00017-X

Henry, L. M., Steele, E. H., Watson, K. H., Bettis, A. H., Gruhn, M., Dunbar, J., Reising, M., & Compas, B. E. (2020). Stress exposure and maternal depression as risk factors for symptoms of anxiety and depression in adolescents. *Child Psychiatry and Human Development*, *51*(4), 572–584. https://doi.org/10.1007/s10578-019-00940-2

Hu, L., & Bentler, P. M. (1999). Cutoff criteria for fit indexes in covariance structure analysis: Conventional criteria versus new alternatives. *Structural Equation Modeling: A Multidisciplinary Journal*, *6*(1), 1–55. https://doi.org/10.1080/10705519909540118

Jacobs, R. H., Reinecke, M. A., Gollan, J. K., & Kane, P. (2008). Empirical evidence of cognitive vulnerability for depression among children and adolescents: A cognitive science and developmental perspective. *Clinical Psychology Review*, *28*(5), 759–782. https://doi.org/10.1016/j.cpr.2007.10.006

Jaycox, L. H., Stein, B. D., Paddock, S., Miles, J. N. V., Chandra, A., Meredith, L. S., Tanielian, T., Hickey, S., & Burnam, M. A. (2009). Impact of teen depression on academic, social, and physical functioning. *Pediatrics*, *124*(4), e596–e605. https://doi.org/10.1542/peds.2008-3348

Kam, C.-M., Greenberg, M. T., Bierman, K. L., Coie, J. D., Dodge, K. A., Foster, M. E., Lochman, J. E., McMahon, R. J., & Pinderhughes, E. E. (2011). Maternal depressive symptoms and child social preference during the early school years: Mediation by maternal warmth and child emotion regulation. *Journal of Abnormal Child Psychology*, *39*(3), 365–377. https://doi.org/10.1007/s10802-010-9468-0

Kessler, R. C., Avenevoli, S., & Merikangas, K. R. (2001). Mood disorders in children and adolescents: An epidemiologic perspective. *Biological Psychiatry*, *49*(12), 1002–1014. https://doi.org/10.1016/s0006-3223(01)01129-5

Khan, S., Gagné, M., Yang, L., & Shapka, J. (2016). Exploring the relationship between adolescents' self-concept and their offline and online social worlds. *Computers in Human Behavior*, *55*, 940–945. https://doi.org/10.1016/j.chb.2015.09.046

Kochanska, G. (2002). Mutually responsive orientation between mothers and their young children: A context for the early development of conscience. *Current Directions in Psychological Science*, *11*(6), 191–195. https://doi.org/10.1111/1467-8721.00198

Kochel, K. P., Ladd, G. W., & Rudolph, K. D. (2012). Longitudinal associations among youth depressive symptoms, peer victimization, and low peer acceptance: An interpersonal process perspective. *Child Development*, *83*(2), 637–650. https://doi.org/10.1111/j.1467-8624.2011.01722.x

Koestner, R., Franz, C., & Weinberger, J. (1990). The family origins of empathic concern: A 26-year longitudinal study. *Journal of Personality and Social Psychology*, *58*(4), 709–717.

Krahé, B., & Möller, I. (2004). Playing violent electronic games, hostile attributional style, and aggression-related norms in German adolescents. *Journal of Adolescence*, *27*(1), 53–69. https://doi.org/10.1016/j.adolescence.2003.10.006

Ladd, G. W., & Pettit, G. S. (2002). Parents and children's peer relations. In M. H. Bornstein (Ed.), *Handbook of parenting. Vol. 5: Practical issues in parenting* (2nd ed., pp. 269–309). Erlbaum.

Ladd, G. W., Birch, S. H., & Buhs, E. S. (1999). Children's social and scholastic lives in kindergarten: Related spheres of influence? *Child Development*, *70*(6), 1373–1400. https://doi.org/10.1111/1467-8624.00101

Laursen, B., & Hartl, A. C. (2013). Understanding loneliness during adolescence: Developmental changes that increase the risk of perceived social isolation. *Journal of Adolescence*, *36*(6), 1261–1268. https://doi.org/10.1016/j.adolescence.2013.06.003

Leung, K., Brew, F. P., Zhang, Z.-X., & Zhang, Y. (2011). Harmony and conflict: A cross-cultural investigation in China and Australia. *Journal of Cross-Cultural Psychology, 42*(5), 795–816. https://doi.org/10.1177/0022022110363474

Lieb, R., Isensee, B., Höfler, M., Pfister, H., & Wittchen, H. (2002). Parental major depression and the risk of depression and other mental disorders in offspring - A prospective-longitudinal community study. *Archives of General Psychiatry, 59*(4), 365–374. https://doi.org/10.1001/archpsyc.59.4.365.

Little, T. D., Cunningham, W. A., Shahar, G., & Widaman, K. F. (2002). To parcel or not to parcel: Exploring the question, weighing the merits. *Structural Equation Modeling: A Multidisciplinary Journal, 9*(2), 151–173. https://doi.org/10.1207/S15328007SEM0902_1

López-López, J. A., Kwong, A. S. F., Washbrook, L., Tilling, K., Fazel, M. S., & Pearson, R. M. (2021). Depressive symptoms and academic achievement in UK adolescents: A cross-lagged analysis with genetic covariates. *Journal of Affective Disorders, 284*, 104–113. https://doi.org/10.1016/j.jad.2021.01.091

Lovejoy, M. C., Graczyk, P. A., O'Hare, E., & Neuman, G. (2000). Maternal depression and parenting behavior. *Clinical Psychology Review, 20*(5), 561–592. https://doi.org/10.1016/S0272-7358(98)00100-7

Lovibond, S. H., & Lovibond, P. F. (1995). *Manual for the depression anxiety stress scales* (2nd ed.). Psychology Foundation, Sydney.

Mazefsky, C. A., Anderson, R., Conner, C. M., & Minshew, N. (2011). Child behavior checklist scores for school-aged children with autism: Preliminary evidence of patterns suggesting the need for referral. *Journal of Psychopathology and Behavioral Assessment, 33*(1), 31–37. https://doi.org/10.1007/s10862-010-9198-1

McDonald, K. L., Bowker, J. C., Rubin, K. H., Laursen, B., & Duchene, M. S. (2010). Interactions between rejection sensitivity and supportive relationships in the prediction of adolescents' internalizing difficulties. *Journal of Youth and Adolescence, 39*(5), 563–574. https://doi.org/10.1007/s10964-010-9519-4

Mennen, F. E., Negriff, S., Schneiderman, J. U., & Trickett, P. K. (2018). Longitudinal associations of maternal depression and adolescents' depression and behaviors: Moderation by maltreatment and sex. *Journal of Family Psychology : JFP : Journal of the Division of Family Psychology of the American Psychological Association (Division 43), 32*(2), 240–250. https://doi.org/10.1037/fam0000394

Möller, I., & Krahé, B. (2009). Exposure to violent video games and aggression in German adolescents: A longitudinal analysis. *Aggressive Behavior, 35*(1), 75–89. https://doi.org/10.1002/ab.20290

Murphy, B. A., Costello, T. H., Watts, A. L., Cheong, Y. F., Berg, J. M., & Lilienfeld, S. O. (2020). Strengths and weaknesses of two empathy measures: A comparison of the measurement precision, construct validity, and incremental validity of two multidimensional indices. *Assessment, 27*(2), 246–260. https://doi.org/10.1177/1073191118777636

Muthén, L. K., & Muthén, B. O. (1998–2015). *Mplus user's guide* (7th ed.). Muthén & Muthén.

Nansel, T. R., Overpeck, M., Pilla, R. S., Ruan, W., Simons-Morton, B., & Scheidt, P. (2001). Bullying behaviors among US youth: Prevalence and association with psychosocial adjustment. *JAMA, 285*(16), 2094–2100. https://doi.org/10.1001/jama.285.16.2094

Patterson, G. R., & Capaldi, D. M. (1990). A mediational model for boys' depressed mood. In J. E. Rolf, A. Masten, D. Ciccheti, K. Neuchterlein, & S. Weintraub (Eds.), *Risk and protective factors in the development of psychopathology* (pp. 141–163). Cambridge University Press.

Platt, B., Kadosh, K. C., & Lau, J. Y. F. (2013). The role of peer rejection in adolescent depression. *Depression and Anxiety, 30*(9), 809–821. https://doi.org/10.1002/da.22120

Roeser, R. W., Midgley, C., & Urdan, T. C. (1996). Perceptions of the school psychological environment and early adolescents' psychological and behavioral functioning in school: The mediating role of goals and belonging. *Journal of Educational Psychology, 88*(3), 408–422. https://doi.org/10.1037/0022-0663.88.3.408

Rogers, W. M., & Schmitt, N. (2004). Parameter recovery and model fit using multidimensional composites: A comparison of four empirical parceling algorithms. *Multivariate Behavioral Research, 39*(3), 379–412. https://doi.org/10.1207/S15327906MBR3903_1

Rohrer, L. M., Cicchetti, D., Rogosch, F. A., Toth, S. L., & Maughan, A. (2011). Effects of maternal negativity and of early and recent recurrent depressive disorder on children's false belief understanding. *Developmental Psychology*, *47*(1), 170–181. https://doi.org/10.1037/a0021305

Scherer, E., Hagaman, A., Chung, E., Rahman, A., O'Donnell, K., & Maselko, J. (2019). The relationship between responsive caregiving and Child outcomes: Evidence from direct observations of mother-child dyads in Pakistan. *BMC Public Health*, *19*(1), Article 252 (2019). https://doi.org/10.1186/s12889-019-6571-1

Siu, A. M., & Shek, D. T. (2005). Validation of the interpersonal reactivity index in a Chinese context. *Research on Social Work Practice*, *15*(2), 118–126. https://doi.org/10.1177/1049731504270384

Spilt, J. L., Van Lier, P. A., C., Leflot, G., Onghena, P., & Colpin, H. (2014). Children's social self-concept and internalizing problems: The influence of peers and teachers. *Child Development*, *85*(3), 1248–1256.

Taylor, A. B., MacKinnon, D. P., & Tein, J. Y. (2008). Tests of the three-path mediated effect. *Organizational Research Methods*, *11*(2), 241–269. https://doi.org/10.1177/1094428107300344

The National Bureau of Statistics of the People's Republic of China. (2018). *China statistical yearbook 2018*. https://www.stats.gov.cn/tjsj/ndsj/2018/indexeh.htm

Trigueros, R., Sanchez-Sanchez, E., Mercader, I., Aguilar-Parra, J. M., López-Liria, R., Morales-Gázquez, M. J., Fernández-Campoy, J. M., & Rocamora, P. (2020). Relationship between emotional intelligence, social skills and peer harassment. A study with high school students. *International Journal of Environmental Research and Public Health*, *17*(12), 4208. https://doi.org/10.3390/ijerph17124208

Tully, E. C., & Donohue, M. R. (2017). Empathic responses to mother's emotions predict internalizing problems in children of depressed mothers. *Child Psychiatry and Human Development*, *48*(1), 94–106.

Vaske, J., Makarios, M., Boisvert, D., Beaver, K. M., & Wright, J. P. (2009). The interaction of drd2 and violent victimization on depression: An analysis by gender and race. *Journal of Affective Disorders*, *112*(1-3), 120–125.

Verboom, C. E., Sijtsema, J. J., Verhulst, F. C., Penninx, B. W. J. H., & Ormel, J. (2014). Longitudinal associations between depressive problems, academic performance, and social functioning in adolescent boys and girls. *Developmental Psychology*, *50*(1), 247–257.

Wang, Y., & Dix, T. (2015). Mother's early depressive symptoms predict children's low social competence in first grade: Mediation by children's social cognition. *Journal of Child Psychology and Psychiatry*, *56*(2), 183–192. https://doi.org/10.1111/jcpp.12297

Witvliet, M., Brendgen, M., van Lier, P. A., Koot, H. M., & Vitaro, F. (2010). Early adolescent depressive symptoms: Prediction from clique isolation, loneliness, and perceived social acceptance. *Journal of Abnormal Child Psychology*, *38*(8), 1045–1056.

Xing, X. P., Wang, M. F., Zhang, Q., He, X. R., & Zhang, W. X. (2011). Gender differences in the reciprocal relationships between parental physical aggression and children's externalizing problem behavior in China. *Journal of Family Psychology : JFP : Journal of the Division of Family Psychology of the American Psychological Association (Division 43)*, *25*(5), 699–708.

Yang, C. M., Nay, S., & Hoyle, R. H. (2010). Three approaches to using lengthy ordinal scales in structural equation models: Parceling, latent scoring, and shortening scales. *Applied Psychological Measurement*, *34*(2), 122–142.

Yang, Y. Q., Chen, L., Ji, L. Q., & Zhang, W. X. (2017). The intergenerational transmission of maternal depression: The mediating role of mother-adolescent relationship and the moderating role of adolescents' negative affectivity. *Psychological Development and Education*, *33*(3), 368–377. https://doi.org/10.16187/j.cnki.issn1001-4918.2017.03.15

Zahn-Waxler, C., & Kochanska, G. (1988). The origins of guilt. *Nebraska Symposium on Motivation. Nebraska Symposium on Motivation*, *36*(1), 183–258.

Zahn-Waxler, C., & Radke-Yarrow, M. (1990). The origins of empathic concern. *Motivation and Emotion*, *14*(2), 107–130. https://doi.org/10.1007/BF00991639

Zahn-Waxler, C., Kochanska, G., Krupnick, J., & McKnew, D. (1990). Patterns of guilt in children of depressed and well mothers. *Developmental Psychology*, *26*(1), 51–59. https://doi.org/10.1037/0012-1649.26.1.51

Zhang, F., You, Z., Fan, C., Gao, C., Cohen, R., Hsueh, Y., & Zhou, Z. (2014). Friendship quality, social preference, proximity prestige, and self-perceived social competence: Interactive influences on children's loneliness. *Journal of School Psychology*, *52*(5), 511–526.

Zhang, W., Li, X., Chen, G., & Cao, Y. (2021). The relationship between positive parenting and adolescent prosocial behavior: The mediating role of empathy and the moderating role of the oxytocin receptor gene. *Acta Psychologica Sinica*, *53*(9), 976–991. https://doi.org/10.3724/SP.J.1041.2021.00976

Zigmond, A. S., & Snaith, R. P. (1983). The hospital anxiety and depression scale. *Acta Psychiatrica Scandinavica*, *67*(6), 361–370. https://doi.org/10.1111/j.1600-0447.1983.tb09716.x

Contributors to Women's Perceived Stress at the Start of Assisted Reproductive Technology

Vera Skvirsky, Orit Taubman – Ben-Ari, Shirley Ben Shlomo, Joseph Azuri and Eran Horowitz

ABSTRACT

Clinicians are often called upon to treat the stress that accompanies Assisted Reproductive Technology (ART). In this study, we sought to examine the contribution of the internal resources of meaning in life and attachment style and the interpersonal resource of self-disclosure to her mother to a woman's level of perceived stress upon commencement of ART. In addition, we examined the association between age and perceived stress. The sample consisted of 180 Israeli women (106 aged 20–34; 74 aged 35–44) who completed a series of self-report questionnaires after their initial meeting with a fertility specialist. Regression analysis indicated that older age, lower attachment anxiety, higher perception of meaning in life, and greater self-disclosure to the mother were related to lower levels of perceived stress. Self-disclosure was also found to mediate the association between avoidant attachment and stress. The study highlights the importance of a woman's personal and interpersonal resources for reducing the experience of stress in the early stages of ART. The results have practical implications for the development of professional interventions seeking to enhance these resources among women embarking on fertility treatment.

It is estimated that 9% of the world's population suffers from infertility (Boivin, Bunting, Collins, & Nygren, 2007), defined as "the failure to achieve a successful pregnancy after 12 months or more of appropriate, unprotected intercourse or therapeutic donor insemination" (Practice Committee of the American Society for Reproductive Medicine, 2013, p. 63). The innate biological need to procreate, coupled with cultural expectations, not only induce more than 50% of couples with fertility issues to seek medical assistance (Boivin et al., 2007) but also render infertility a stressful experience that arouses distress, anxiety, and feelings of loss, failure, and pain (Berger, Paul, & Henshaw, 2013; Domar & Gross, 2012; Ying, Wu, & Loke, 2015). However, while ART may help in overcoming the physiological problems, it is also likely to elevate the level of distress (Greil, McQuillan, Lowry, & Shreffler, 2011). This is where clinicians may intervene to help individuals and couples to cope.

Moreover, although findings are inconsistent, some studies indicate that stress may negatively affect the likelihood of conception (Buck Louis et al., 2011; Lynch, Sundaram, Maisog, Sweeney, & Buck Louis, 2014), and that women with fertility issues who have lower levels of stress are more apt to seek and remain in treatment (Brandes et al., 2009). Thus, it seems highly important, from both the medical and the psychological perspectives, to delve deeper into the factors which may impact perceived stress in the early stages of ART.

The moment in a woman's life at which she turns to a fertility clinic is marked by a high level of uncertainty. Such women have typically experienced a history of failure to conceive or bring a pregnancy to term, implying a baseline level of stress (Domar & Gross, 2012). The initial consultation with a specialist is meant to deepen the woman's knowledge of infertility and ART, and indeed, one study found that the level of anxiety decreased following this consultation (Childress et al., 2015). However, in another study women were shown to exhibit the same level of emotional distress (especially anxiety) prior to their first fertility clinic appointment and six months later (Anderson, Sharpe, Rattray, & Irvine, 2003). Psychosocial interventions for women (and men) at this point in their lives might play an important role in reducing their level of stress.

Lazarus and Folkman's (1984) model of stress and coping maintains that when individuals experience stress, they make consistent cognitive and behavioral efforts to restore balance in light of the new external and/or internal demands on their resources, whether physical, social, or psychological. Successful coping therefore depends on the resources available to them. On this basis, the present study sought to identify resources, both internal (meaning in life, attachment style) and interpersonal (tendency for self-disclosure to the mother), that may contribute to the level of perceived stress of women following their initial contact with a fertility specialist. Although studies of infertility generally refer to the couple dyad, as by definition, infertility affects the lives of both partners (Benyamini, Gozlan, & Kokia, 2009; Ying et al., 2015), several investigations have highlighted the importance of the family's support to the woman (High & Steuber, 2014; Vassard, Lund, Pinborg, Boivin, & Schmidt, 2012). With this in mind, we chose to turn the spotlight on the mother–daughter relationship, another major dyad in a woman's life and one that has received very little research attention.

Furthermore, as individuals are innately driven to find meaning and significance in their lives (Frankl, 1963), ***meaning in life*** is a crucial component of human experience. Global meaning in life has been defined as "the sense made of, and significance felt regarding, the nature of one's being and existence" (Steger, Frazier, Oishi, & Kaler, 2006, p. 81). In everyday life, global meaning informs individuals' understanding of themselves and their lives and directs their personal projects and, through them, their general sense of well-being and life satisfaction (Steger, 2009; Steger et al., 2006). The search for meaning in life is an independent dimension, which does not imply an absence of meaning, but rather refers to the drive and orientation to find meaning (Steger et al., 2006). Presence of meaning in life has been related to higher well-being, life satisfaction, and positive emotions, as well as lower depression, distress, and negative emotions. The search for meaning has been associated with lower well-being and higher depression (Dezutter, Luyckx, & Wachholtz, 2015; Steger et al., 2006; Steger, Oishi, & Kashdan, 2009). Both components have been shown to be relatively stable across time, suggesting that meaning in life is a stable intrapersonal resource (Dezutter et al., 2015; Steger & Kashdan, 2007).

A study of women treated with IVF found some degree of uncertainty regarding the meaning of life (Su, Chen, Chen, Yang, & Hung, 2006). On the other hand, Mosalanejad and Koolee (2013) found that group logotherapy treatment, which focuses on meaning in life, decreased worry and perceived stress perception among women coping with infertility.

Another important resource is ***attachment orientation*** (Bowlby, 1973), which shapes the way people cope with and adjust to stressful events, and has been conceptualized as an emotion regulation device that governs an individual's emotional responses (Mikulincer & Shaver, 2007). Current literature generally refers to two dimensions of insecure attachment: avoidance and anxiety. People who score low on both dimensions are considered to have a secure attachment style, which is reflected in a global sense of security, trust in others, comfort with closeness and interdependence, and constructive coping with threats and stressors (Mikulincer & Shaver, 2007). Attachment anxiety is characterized by a fear of interpersonal rejection or abandonment, a tendency to focus on distress, rumination on negative thoughts, and the adoption of emotion-focused coping strategies, all of which exacerbate, rather than diminish, distress. Attachment avoidance is characterized by fear of dependence and interpersonal intimacy, and by distancing oneself cognitively or behaviorally from the source of distress (Shaver & Mikulincer, 2002).

Attachment styles can be an important resource for women coping with infertility. Studies show that securely attached women report higher well-being, less distress, and more dyadic consensus than women with insecure attachment (Mikulincer, Horesh, Levy-Shiff, Manovich, & Shalev, 1998), and that both attachment anxiety and avoidance correlate positively with infertility-related stress in women at different stages of fertility treatment (Bayley, Slade, & Lashen, 2009; Donarelli et al., 2012). Moreover, attachment anxiety was positively associated with pre-IVF distress (Van den Broeck, D'Hooghe, Enzlin, & Demyttenaere, 2010), and women with attachment avoidance were more poorly adjusted to infertility (Mahajan et al., 2008).

The literature also highlights the substantial importance of interpersonal resources. One potential resource of this sort is ***self-disclosure***, a complex and dynamic process of revealing one's thoughts, feelings, and experiences to another person (Dindia, 2002). Self-disclosure may be seen as a self-regulation technique in which individuals translate their emotional experiences into language, thereby helping to construct their response to an emotionally charged situation (Smyth, Pennebaker, & Arigo, 2012). Moreover, emotional self-disclosure is a linchpin connecting various aspects of well-being, positive adjustment, and successful psychotherapeutic treatment (Kahn, Hucke, Bradley, Glinski, & Malak, 2012). For instance, research has shown that experimental emotional self-disclosure may have a beneficial impact on physical health, psychological well-being, and general adjustment (Frattaroli, 2006; Magai, Consedine, Fiori, & King, 2009).

Moreover, self-disclosure is an interpersonal process which is dependent not only on the individual but also on the characteristics of the recipient (Ignatius & Kokkonen, 2007), and may reflect a positive relationship feature of closeness and support (Buhrmester & Furman, 2008). In the current study, we chose to emphasize self-disclosure as an inter-personal resource which characterizes a unique relationship – the mother–daughter dyad. The mother, commonly the primary caregiver for children, is the main object of identification and role model for her daughter throughout her life (Shrier, Tompsett, & Shrier, 2004). Even in adulthood, a woman's mother remains an important source of attachment and support, despite the potential for conflict between the two sides as well (Bernstein, 2004; Bojczyk, Lehan, McWey, Melson, & Kaufman 2011; Notman, 2006). Thus, sharing her thoughts and feelings with this important figure in her life may help to reduce the stress of a woman entering ART. Indeed, research has found that full disclosure of one's fertility status is associated with lower social and personal fertility-related stress (Martins et al., 2013). However, given that infertility is a particularly sensitive topic whose disclosure may also depend on the consent of the spouse (Steuber & Solomon, 2011), the current study focused on a woman's tendency to self-disclose to her mother in general. Furthermore, since avoidant individuals report less inclination to disclose personal feelings or express emotions (Mikulincer & Shaver, 2007), we considered the possibility that self-disclosure to the mother plays a mediating role in the relationship between avoidant attachment style and perceived stress.

The current study

This study therefore sought to identify factors that may impact the level of stress of women embarking on ART. On the basis of the literature, the following hypotheses were formulated:

1. A higher level of presence of meaning in life and a lower level of search for meaning in life will be associated with a lower level of perceived stress.
2. Higher levels of attachment anxiety and avoidance will be associated with a higher level of perceived stress.
3. Higher self-disclosure to the mother will be associated with a lower level of perceived stress.
4. Self-disclosure will mediate the relationship between avoidant attachment style and perceived stress.

In addition, we explored differences between younger (under 35) and older (35 and over) women coping with infertility, as medical research indicates that once a woman has reached her mid-30s, physiological processes in the female body lead to a decrease in fertility and ovarian function and a rise in the length of time required to conceive. The age of 35 is considered the cut-off point at which the decline in fertility becomes sharper (Balasch, 2010; Liu et al., 2012).

Method

Procedure

The current study is part of the first phase of an extensive longitudinal investigation approved by the Institutional Review Board of the health provider through which the participants were recruited. Previous articles based on the data generated in Phase 1 of the research project have related to other aspects (Ben Shlomo, Pascal, Taubman - Ben-Ari, Azuri, & Horowtz, 2017; Ben Shlomo, Skvirsky, Taubman - Ben-Ari, Azuri, & Horowitz, 2017; Skvirsky, Taubman - Ben-Ari, Ben Shlomo, Azuri, & Horowitz, in press). The sample consisted of women who arrived for their initial visit at one of three large ART units in Israel. Women were included in the study if they were in the first phase of fertility consultation and could understand and complete questionnaires in Hebrew. We placed no restrictions on age, education, or socioeconomic status. The doctor in charge of the unit approached the participants, explained the purpose of the study, and assured the women that their participation was in no way related to the medical treatment they would receive at the clinic. After giving their written consent to participate in the study, the women received the questionnaire in a sealed envelope, along with a stamped self-addressed envelope in which to return it. Subsequently, the administrative director of the study (a clinical social worker) contacted the women to verify that the questionnaire had been completed and returned, and to respond to any distress it may have aroused.

Participants

During the data collection period, 269 women met the inclusion criteria (i.e., they were in the initial phase of ART and were capable of completing the Hebrew instruments). Eighteen women declined to participate. Of the 251 who agreed to take part in the study, 189 (75.3%) completed the questionnaire in full. As one of the issues investigated in the current study was self-disclosure to the mother, 9 women whose mothers had passed away were excluded from the sample.

The final sample consisted of 180 women aged 20–44 ($M = 32.96$, $SD = 5.24$), 106 in the "younger" age group (below 35; $M = 29.25$, $SD = 3.12$) and 74 in the "older" group (35 and over; $M = 38.28$, $SD = 2.20$). In the majority of cases, infertility was due to a condition in the female (34.4%) or to unexplained infertility (30.6%). In 18.9%, it was due to male factor infertility, and in 5.0% to conditions in both partners. The remaining 7.2% consisted of women who were requesting sperm donation for personal reasons. About half the women (54.4%) experienced secondary infertility (difficulty conceiving after having previously conceived, whether leading to abortion, miscarriage, or normal pregnancy), and 42.8% primary infertility (having never been able to conceive). No information was provided about the source of infertility for seven women and about the type of infertility for five. The large majority of participants (90.6%) were married or in a stable relationship. Most reported very good or good health (92.2%), academic education (67.8%), and average income (72.8%). Ninety-seven participants had no children, and 83 were already mothers (generally 1–2 children, $M = 1.63$, $SD = 1.08$).

Instruments

The *Perceived Stress Scale* (PSS; Cohen, Kamarck, & Mermelstein, 1983), a 13-item scale, was used to assess the woman's subjective perception of her level of stress in this period in her life (e.g., "How often have you been upset because of something that happened unexpectedly?"). Responses were given on a scale ranging from 1 (*never*) to 4 (*often*).

As the internal reliability of the scale was adequate (Cronbach's alpha = 0.83), a total score was computed averaging the responses to all items, with higher scores indicating greater stress.

The *Meaning in Life Questionnaire* (MLQ; Steger et al., 2006) was used to measure the two dimensions of this internal resource. The instrument consists of two 5-item subscales, one assessing the search for meaning in life (e.g., "I am searching for meaning in my life"; Cronbach's alpha =0.87), and the other the presence of meaning in life (e.g., "I understand my life's meaning"; Cronbach's alpha =0.84). Responses were marked on a scale ranging from 1 (*absolutely untrue*) to 7 (*absolutely true*). Two meaning in life scores were computed for each participant by averaging her responses to the items on each subscale, with higher scores indicating greater search for meaning or presence of meaning.

Experiences in Close Relationships Scale - Short Form (ECR-S; Brennan, Clark, & Shaver, 1998; Mikulincer & Shaver, 2007) was used to assess attachment style. The scale consists of 18 items, 9 tapping attachment anxiety (e.g., "I do not often worry about being abandoned"), and 9 tapping attachment avoidance (e.g., "I try to avoid getting too close to others"). Two items were removed, one from each subscale, as they reduced the reliability of the scale. The final Cronbach's alphas were 0.74 for anxious attachment, and 0.69 for avoidant attachment. Responses were marked on a scale ranging from 1 (*strongly disagree*) to 7 (*strongly agree*). Two attachment orientation scores were computed for each participant by averaging her responses to the items on each dimension, with higher scores indicating greater anxious or avoidant attachment.

The *Self-Disclosure Index* (SDI; Miller, Berg, & Archer, 1983), a 10-item scale, was adapted to measure the tendency of women to disclose their thoughts and feelings to their mothers (e.g., "I tell my mother about my deepest feelings"; "I tell my mother about my worst fears"). Responses were given on a scale ranging from 1 (*discuss not at all*) to 6 (*discuss fully and completely*). As the internal reliability of the scale was high (Cronbach's alpha =0.95), a total score was computed by averaging the responses to all items, with a higher score indicating the woman's greater tendency to self-disclose to her mother.

A demographic questionnaire was used to obtain information regarding personal and family characteristics, including age, education (primary/secondary/post-secondary/academic), physical health status (very poor/poor/average/good/very good), economic status (below average/average/above average), marital status (single/married/divorced/unmarried couple), and whether or not the woman already had children and if so, how many. The fertility doctor provided data regarding primary/secondary infertility and the source of infertility.

Data Analysis

In the first stage of analysis, we conducted *t*-tests for independent samples to examine differences between the women in the two age groups (below 35, 35 and over). Next, we addressed the issue of missing values due to incomplete questionnaires since it may cause biased sampling. Analysis across the research variables revealed relatively low rates of missing values, ranging from as low as none to a high of 2.8 percent. Little's test for

Table 1. Means, Standard Deviations, and *t*-Tests for the Study Variables, by Age Group.

	Younger women ($n = 106$)		Older women ($n = 74$)		
	M	SD	M	SD	*t*
Perceived stress	2.34	0.43	2.26	0.41	1.20
Search for meaning in life	4.51	1.19	4.15	1.39	1.89
Presence of meaning in life	5.12	0.96	5.22	0.93	−0.73
Attachment anxiety	2.91	1.09	2.83	0.91	0.49
Attachment avoidance	2.88	0.90	2.79	0.91	0.71
Self-disclosure to the mother	3.95	1.20	3.32	1.26	3.34***

***$p \leq 0.001$.

MCAR revealed that missing items were completely at random (Chi-Square = 64.28, df = 78, $p = 0.868$), and that no missing values were related to a specific variable or a specific respondent (Little, 1988). A multiple imputation procedure (SPSS V.21), using a stochastic regression model to impute random values for the missing values based on prior information about the data (Enders, 2010), was then conducted. When the rate of missing values is low, or less than five percent across all variables, as it was in our case, a single imputed repeat is considered sufficient (Little, 2013, p.55). In the next stage, we computed Pearson correlations to examine the associations between the independent variables (attachment style, meaning in life, self-disclosure to the mother), and the outcome variable of perceived stress. In the fourth stage of analysis, we performed a hierarchical regression to examine the unique and combined contribution of the independent variables to women's perception of stress. In light of the literature, variables were entered in a forced order. The background characteristics (age group, primary/secondary infertility, education, economic status, physical health status, and marital status) were entered in Step 1. The cause of infertility was not included in this step following a Chi-Square test which yielded an association between marital status and the cause of infertility ($\chi^2(1) = 10.38$, $p < 0.001$): sperm donation was reported by 1.3% of married/in a relationship women, and by 73.3% of single women. Moreover, an ANOVA showed no association between the cause of infertility and perceived stress. Thus, in the further statistical analysis we controlled for marital status and not for the cause of infertility. We also chose to enter the type of infertility and not whether women already had children for two reasons. First, the two variables were strongly correlated ($r = -0.79$, $p = 0.00$), and secondly, previous research has shown that women who have never conceived differ from women who have conceived, regardless of the outcome of the previous conception (Greil, Johnson, McQuillan, & Lacy, 2011). The internal resources (attachment style, meaning in life) were entered in Step 2, and the interpersonal resource (self-disclosure to the mother) in Step 3, with R^2 used to assess the model's fit. Finally, to test our fourth hypothesis regarding the potential mediation of self-disclosure in the link between avoidant attachment style and perceived stress, PROCESS analysis (Hayes, 2013), examining direct and indirect effects, was performed.

Results

No significant differences in sociodemographic characteristics were found between the two age groups, save for the fact that more women in the "older" group had children,

Table 2. Hierarchical Regression Coefficients (Beta Weights) for Perceived Stress at the Start of Fertility Treatment ($N = 180$).

	β	t	ΔR^2
Step 1			0.10**
Age group	−0.16	−1.97*	
Primary/secondary infertility	−0.07	−0.90	
Education	−0.11	−1.50	
Economic status	−0.03	−0.36	
Health status	−0.24	−3.29***	
Marital status	−0.09	−1.11	
Step 2			0.15***
Attachment anxiety	0.22	3.07**	
Attachment avoidance	−0.03	−0.40	
Search for meaning in life	0.03	0.36	
Presence of meaning in life	−0.31	−4.25***	
Step 3			0.02*
Self-disclosure to the mother	−0.17	−2.31*	
R^2			0.27***
F (11, 168)			5.60

*$p \leq 0.05$, **$p < 0.01$, ***$p \leq 0.001$.

were characterized by secondary infertility, and were single and therefore asking for a sperm donation. These differences were controlled for in the statistical analyses.

The results of the t-tests performed to identify differences between the groups on the study variables appear in Table 1. As can be seen from the table, younger women reported a higher level of self-disclosure than older women. No significant differences were found between the two groups on any of the other variables.

Pearson correlations examining associations between the variables revealed a significant positive correlation between women's perceived stress and attachment anxiety ($r = 0.27$, $p = 0.00$), but not attachment avoidance ($r = 0.07$, $p = 0.34$). Thus, higher attachment anxiety was associated with higher stress. In addition, a significant negative correlation was found between perceived stress and presence of meaning in life ($r = -0.38$, $p = 0.00$), but not the search for meaning ($r = 0.06$, $p = 0.44$). Thus, the higher the presence of meaning in life, the lower the level of stress the woman perceived. Another significant, albeit weak, negative correlation was found between the tendency for self-disclosure and perceived stress ($r = -0.16$, $p = 0.03$), indicating that the more a woman discloses her feelings and thoughts to her mother, the less stress she tends to experience.

Table 2 presents the results of the regression analysis, revealing that the variables explained 27% of the variance in perceived stress. The sociodemographic characteristics in Step 1 accounted for 10% of the explained variance, with older women and women in better health reporting lower levels of stress. The internal resources in Step 2 contributed a further 15% to the explanation of the variance, showing that lower attachment anxiety and higher perception of presence of meaning in life were associated with lower levels of perceived stress. In Step 3, a woman's tendency to self-disclose to her mother contributed another 2% to the explained variance, with higher self-disclosure related to lower levels of perceived stress at the beginning of ART.

The PROCESS analysis (Hayes, 2013) yielded the predicted indirect effect, with self-disclosure fully mediating the relationship between avoidant attachment style and perceived stress (ind =0.02, $p < 0.05$, 95% CI [0.003,0.06]). In other words, higher avoidant attachment was associated with lower self-disclosure ($b = -0.42$, $p = 0.00$), which, in turn, was associated with a higher perception of stress ($b = -0.06$, $p = 0.02$). The direct effect between avoidant attachment and perceived stress was insignificant ($b = -0.04$, $p = 0.27$).

Discussion

Relying on Lazarus and Folkman's model of stress and coping (1984), the current study examined the role of the internal resources of meaning in life and attachment orientation and the interpersonal resource of disclosure to the mother in reducing the perceived stress of a woman at the start of ART. As predicted, the presence of meaning in life was associated with less perceived stress. This is in line with previous studies indicating that people who perceive meaning in their life are less depressed and have more positive affect and greater satisfaction with their lives (Steger et al., 2006). Thus, in spite of the difficulties to conceive, women who consider their lives meaningful in general may experience less stress. However, although we expected the search for meaning in life to be associated with a higher level of stress, no such association emerged. This may be due to the nature of this dimension. Since the search for meaning does not necessarily imply the absence of it, it is possible that women scoring high on this variable are seeking to add to their current sources of meaning or to deepen their understanding of the meaning they already perceive (Steger et al., 2006). Nevertheless, the finding of a link between presence of meaning and a lower level of stress suggests that women entering ART may benefit from interventions aimed at helping them find new or enhanced meaning in life beyond the role of motherhood, particularly as a highly stressful event may impact an individual's global sense of the meaningfulness of life (Park, 2010).

Also in line with our hypothesis, as well as with previous studies (Donarelli et al., 2012; Van den Broeck et al., 2010), high attachment anxiety was associated with higher perceived stress. Contrary to expectations, however, no direct association emerged between attachment avoidance and stress. This may stem from the fact that avoidant persons tend to cope with painful emotions by means of denial or suppression (Mikulincer & Shaver, 2007), thus concealing their stress.

Furthermore, as predicted, self-disclosure to the mother was associated with a lower perception of stress, indicating that self-disclosure may function as a positive coping strategy. In addition, since self-disclosure relies on closeness between the two individuals, particularly in such a sensitive situation as infertility (Steuber & Solomon, 2011), the mother may be a unique resource for women about to undergo fertility treatment. This appears to be especially true for younger women, who were found to disclose more to their mothers than older women. It may reflect that younger women, feel more comfortable in sharing their feelings with their mothers, and may depend more on this relationship, and the support provided by their mothers, as was also found in a previous study (Skvirsky et al., in press). Moreover, in confirmation of our hypothesis, self-disclosure mediated the association between avoidant attachment and perceived stress, indicating that women high on avoidant attachment tend to self-disclose less, which, in turn, was associated with higher stress. This finding also accords with attachment theory, which holds that avoidant people refrain from disclosing their personal feelings or emotions (Mikulincer & Shaver, 2007), which may make them more vulnerable to stress.

Two additional variables were found to play a role in the level of perceived stress of women following their initial consultation at a fertility clinic: physical health and age. It is not surprising that women with better physical health reported lower levels of stress, since good health has consistently been related to psychological well-being and happiness (Baumeister, Vohs, Aaker, & Garbinsky, 2013). The finding that younger women reported higher levels of perceived stress is less expected, as from the medical point of view, they have a better chance of conceiving. From a psychological perspective, however, this finding may reflect the fact that women aged 35 and over are less dismayed by fertility problems, as age is a well-known risk factor. In contrast, younger women may not expect to encounter difficulties achieving pregnancy, and thus may experience more stress. Interestingly, other demographic variables (education, economic and marital status, primary/secondary infertility) were not associated with stress. It is possible that at this early stage of ART, these variables do not yet come into play.

Certain limitations of the study should be noted. First, it relies solely on self-report instruments since we were interested in tapping women's personal feelings. However, future studies might attempt to corroborate self-reports by approaching people close to the woman, such as her mother or partner. Secondly, this was a cross-sectional study conducted at a single point in time, a fact that impeded determination of the temporal sequence of stress and infertility. It might be worthwhile for future studies to adopt a longitudinal design to examine the contribution of the resources investigated here to the trajectory of women's stress over the course of fertility treatment.

Despite these limitations, the study has several strengths. By questioning women on their very first visit to a fertility clinic, it shows that stress already exists at this early stage, and thus clinicians should be aware of this issue and address it. In addition, it indicates that higher attachment anxiety and lower perception of meaning in life are related to higher stress, thereby suggesting possible avenues for reducing the stress of women at the initial stage of treatment. Moreover, in contrast to the customary reference to the couple dyad, the study explored the role of the mother-daughter dyad, revealing it to be an important resource for women at this point in their lives. This finding affords clinicians an opportunity to expand their traditional perception of the spouse as the woman's main source of support. Finally, the study indicates the relevance of age not only from a physiological standpoint, but also from a psychological perspective.

Theoretical and Practical Implications

The results of the study suggest the importance of professional interventions aimed specifically at women embarking on ART. By reducing the level of stress experienced at this early stage, such interventions can not only improve women's psychological well-being, but may also enhance the chance of the treatment's success. The study indicates that the design of these interventions should relate differentially to younger and older women, and should also take into account their attachment style. In addition, they might try to incorporate methods that focus on enhancing the presence of meaning in life. Furthermore, as the study shows that the mother can play a role in reducing the woman's level of stress; interventions might consider the possibility of promoting a closer mother-- daughter relationship, or including the mother as a partner in the process.

References

Anderson, K. M., Sharpe, M., Rattray, A., & Irvine, D. S. (2003). Distress and concerns in couples referred to a specialist infertility clinic. *Journal of Psychosomatic Research*, *54*(4), 353–355. doi:10.1016/S0022-3999(02)00398-7

Balasch, J. (2010). Ageing and infertility: An overview. *Gynecological Endocrinology, 26*(12), 855–860. doi:10.3109/09513590.2010.501889

Baumeister, R. F., Vohs, K. D., Aaker, J. L., & Garbinsky, E. N. (2013). Some key differences between a happy life and a meaningful life. *The Journal of Positive Psychology, 8*(6), 505–516. doi:10.1080/17439760.2013.830764

Bayley, T. M., Slade, P., & Lashen, H. (2009). Relationships between attachment, appraisal, coping and adjustment in men and women experiencing infertility concerns. *Human Reproduction, 24*(11), 2827–2837. doi:10.1093/humrep/dep235

Ben Shlomo, S., Pascal, M., Taubman – Ben-Ari, O., Azuri, Y., & Horowtz, E. (2017). Life satisfaction of women in early stages of fertility treatment. *Women & Health, 57*(5), 566–582. doi:10.1080/03630242.2016.1178682

Ben Shlomo, S., Skvirsky, V., Taubman – Ben-Ari, O., Azuri, J., & Horowitz, E. (2017). Mental health of women entering fertility treatment: What role do age and internal resources play? *Stress & Health, 33*(4), 470–476. doi:10.1002/smi.2733

Benyamini, Y., Gozlan, M., & Kokia, E. (2009). Women's and men's perceptions of infertility and their associations with psychological adjustment: A dyadic approach. *British Journal of Health Psychology, 14*(1), 1–16. doi:10.1348/135910708X279288

Berger, R., Paul, M. S., & Henshaw, L. A. (2013). Women's experience of infertility: A multi-systemic perspective. *Journal of International Women's Studies, 14*, 54–68.

Bernstein, P. (2004). Mothers and daughters from today's psychoanalytic perspective. *Psychoanalytic Inquiry, 24*(5), 601–628. doi:10.1080/07351692409349106

Boivin, J., Bunting, L., Collins, J. A., & Nygren, K. G. (2007). International estimates of infertility prevalence and treatment-seeking: Potential need and demand for infertility medical care. *Human Reproduction, 22*(6), 1506–1512. doi:10.1093/humrep/dem046

Bojczyk, K. E., Lehan, T. J., McWey, L. M., Melson, G. F., & Kaufman, D. R. (2011). Mothers' and their adult daughters' perceptions of their relationship. *Journal of Family Issues, 32*(4), 452–481. doi:10.1177/0192513X10384073

Bowlby, J. (1973). *Attachment and loss: Vol. 2. Separation: Anxiety and anger*. New York: Basic Books.

Brandes, M., Van Der Steen, J. O. M., Bokdam, S. B., Hamilton, C. J. C. M., De Bruin, J. P., Nelen, W. L. D. M., & Kremer, J. A. M. (2009). When and why do subfertile couples discontinue their fertility care? A longitudinal cohort study in a secondary care subfertility population. *Human Reproduction, 24*(12), 3127–3135. doi:10.1093/humrep/dep340

Brennan, K. A., Clark, C. L., & Shaver, P. R. (1998). Self-report measurement of adult romantic attachment: An integrative overview. In J.A. Simpson & W.S. Rholes (Eds.), *Attachment theory and close relationships* (pp. 46–76). New York: Guilford Press

Buck Louis, G. M., Lum, K. J., Sundaram, R., Chen, Z., Kim, K. J., Lynch, C. D., … Pyper, C. (2011). Stress reduces conception probabilities across the fertile window: Evidence in support of relaxation. *Fertility and Sterility, 95*(7), 2184–2189. doi:10.1016/j.fertnstert.2010.06.078

Buhrmester, D., & Furman, W. (2008). *The network of relationships inventory: Relationship qualities version*. Unpublished measure, Dallas: University of Texas.

Childress, K. J., Lawson, A. K., Ghant, M. S., Mendoza, G., Cardozo, E. R., Confino, E., & Marsh, E. E. (2015). First contact: The intersection of demographics, knowledge, and appraisal of treatment at the initial infertility visit. *Fertility and Sterility, 104*(1), 180–187. doi:10.1016/j.fertnstert.2015.04.002

Cohen, S., Kamarck, T., & Mermelstein, R. (1983). A global measure of perceived stress. *Journal of Health and Social Behavior, 24*(4), 385–396. doi:10.2307/2136404

Dezutter, J., Luyckx, K., & Wachholtz, A. (2015). Meaning in life in chronic pain patients over time: Associations with pain experience and psychological well-being. *Journal of Behavioral Medicine, 38*(2), 384–396. doi:10.1007/s10865-014-9614-1

Dindia, K. (2002). Self-disclosure research: Knowledge through meta-analysis. In M. Allen, R. W. Preiss, B. M. Gayle, & N. A. Burrell (Eds.), *Interpersonal communication research: Advances through meta-analysis* (pp. 169–185). Mahwah, NJ: Lawrence Erlbaum Associates.

Domar, A., & Gross, J. (2012). Stress and ART. In E.S. Ginsburg & C. Racowsky (Eds.), *In vitro fertilization: A comprehensive guide* (pp. 201–209). New York: Springer.

Donarelli, Z., Lo Coco, G., Gullo, S., Marino, A., Volpes, A., & Allegra, A. (2012). Are attachment dimensions associated with infertility-related stress in couples undergoing their first IVF treatment? A study on the individual and cross-partner effect. *Human Reproduction*, *27*(11), 3215–3225. doi:10.1093/humrep/des307

Enders, C. K. (2010). *Applied missing data analysis*. New York: Guilford.

Frankl, V. E. (1963). *Man's search for meaning: An introduction to logotherapy*. New York: Washington Square Press.

Frattaroli, J. (2006). Experimental disclosure and its moderators: A meta-analysis. *Psychological Bulletin*, *132*(6), 823–865. doi:10.1037/0033-2909.132.6.823

Greil, A. L., Johnson, K. M., McQuillan, J., & Lacy, N. (2011). Are prior pregnancy outcomes relevant for models of fertility-specific distress or infertility helpseeking? *Human Fertility (Cambridge, England)*, *14*(3), 160–166. doi:10.3109/14647273.2011.587229

Greil, A. L., McQuillan, J., Lowry, M., & Shreffler, K. M. (2011). Infertility treatment and fertility-specific distress: A longitudinal analysis of a population-based sample of U.S. women. *Social Science & Medicine*, *73*(1), 87–94. doi:10.1016/j.socscimed.2011.04.023

Hayes, A. F. (2013). *Introduction to mediation, moderation, and conditional process analysis*. New York: Guilford.

High, A. C., & Steuber, K. R. (2014). An examination of support (in)adequacy: Types, sources, and consequences of social support among infertile women. *Communication Monographs*, *81*(2), 157–178. doi:10.1080/03637751.2013.878868

Ignatius, E., & Kokkonen, M. (2007). Factors contributing to verbal self-disclosure. *Nordic Psychology*, *59*(4), 362–391. doi:10.1027/1901-2276.59.4.362

Kahn, J. H., Hucke, B. E., Bradley, A. M., Glinski, A. J., & Malak, B. L. (2012). The Distress Disclosure Index: A research review and multitrait–multimethod examination. *Journal of Counseling Psychology*, *59*(1), 134–149. doi:10.1037/a0025716

Lazarus, R. S., & Folkman, S. (1984). *Stress, appraisal, and coping*. New York: Springer.

Little, R. J. A. (1988). A test of missing completely at random for multivariate data with missing values. *Journal of the American Statistical Association*, *83*(404), 1198–1202. doi:10.1080/01621459.1988.10478722

Little, T. D. (2013). *Longitudinal structural equation modeling*. New York: Guilford.

Liu, K., Case, A., Cheung, A. P., Sierra, S., AlAsiri, S., Carranza-Mamane, B., … Wong, B. C.-M. (2012). Advanced reproductive age and fertility. *International Journal of Gynecology and Obstetrics*, *117*(1), 95–102. doi:10.1016/S1701-2163(16)35087-3

Lynch, C. D., Sundaram, R., Maisog, J. M., Sweeney, A. M., & Buck Louis, G. M. (2014). Preconception stress increases the risk of infertility: Results from a couple-based prospective cohort study—the LIFE study. *Human Reproduction*, *29*(5), 1067–1075. doi:10.1093/humrep/deu032

Magai, C., Consedine, N. S., Fiori, K. L., & King, A. R. (2009). Sharing the good, sharing the bad: The benefits of emotional self-disclosure among middle-aged and older adults. *Journal of Aging and Health*, *21*(2), 286–313. doi:10.1177/0898264308328980

Mahajan, N. N., Turnbull, D. A., Davies, M. J., Jindal, U. N., Briggs, N. E., & Taplin, J. E. (2008). Adjustment to infertility: The role of intrapersonal and interpersonal resources/vulnerabilities. *Human Reproduction*, *24*(4), 906–912. doi:10.1093/humrep/den462

Martins, M. V., Peterson, B. D., Costa, P., Costa, M. E., Lund, R., & Schmidt, L. (2013). Interactive effects of social support and disclosure on fertility-related stress. *Journal of Social and Personal Relationships*, *30*(4), 371–388. doi:10.1177/0265407512456672

Mikulincer, M., Horesh, N., Levy-Shiff, R., Manovich, R., & Shalev, J. (1998). The contribution of adult attachment style to the adjustment to infertility. *British Journal of Medical Psychology*, *71*(3), 265–280. doi:10.1111/j.2044-8341.1998.tb00991.x

Mikulincer, M., & Shaver, P. R. (2007). *Attachment in adulthood: Structure, dynamics, and change*. New York: Guilford.

Miller, L. C., Berg, J. H., & Archer, R. L. (1983). Openers: Individuals who elicit intimate self-disclosure. *Journal of Personality and Social Psychology*, *44*(6), 1234–1244. doi:10.1037/0022-3514.44.6.1234

Mosalanejad, L. K., & Koolee, A. (2013). Looking at infertility treatment through the lens of the meaning of life: The effect of group logotherapy on psychological distress in infertile women. *International Journal of Fertility and Sterility*, *6*, 224–231.

Notman, M. T. (2006). Mothers and daughters as adults. *Psychoanalytic Inquiry*, *26*(1), 137–153. doi:10.1080/07351690609353116

Park, C. L. (2010). Making sense of the meaning literature: An integrative review of meaning making and its effects on adjustment to stressful life events. *Psychological Bulletin*, *136*(2), 257–301. doi:10.1037/a0018301

Practice Committee of the American Society for Reproductive Medicine (2013). Definitions of infertility and recurrent pregnancy loss: A committee opinion. *Fertility and Sterility*, *99*(1), 63. doi:10.1016/j.fertnstert.2012.09.023

Shrier, D. K., Tompsett, M., & Shrier, L. A. (2004). Adult mother–daughter relationships: A review of the theoretical and research literature. *Journal of the American Academy of Psychoanalysis and Dynamic Psychiatry*, *32*(1), 91–115. doi:10.1521/jaap.32.1.91.28332

Shaver, P. R., & Mikulincer, M. (2002). Attachment-related psychodynamics. *Attachment & Human Development*, *4*(2), 133–161. doi:10.1080/14616730210154171

Skvirsky, V., Taubman - Ben-Ari, O., Ben Shlomo, S., Azuri, J., & Horowitz, E. (in press). Are mothers a source of support for women entering fertility treatment? Health Care for Women International. doi:10.1080/07399332.2018.1424170

Smyth, J. M., Pennebaker, J. W., & Arigo, P. (2012). What are the health effects of disclosure?. In A. Baum, T.A. Revenson, & J. Singer (Eds.), *Handbook of health psychology* (2nd ed.) (pp. 175–191). New York: Psychology Press.

Steger, M. F. (2009). Meaning in life. In S.J. Lopez (Ed.), *Oxford handbook of positive psychology* (2nd ed.) (pp. 679–687). Oxford, UK: Oxford University Press.

Steger, M. F., Frazier, P., Oishi, S., & Kaler, M. (2006). The Meaning in Life Questionnaire: Assessing the presence of and search for meaning in life. *Journal of Counseling Psychology*, *53*(1), 80–93. doi:10.1037/0022-0167.53.1.80

Steger, M. F., & Kashdan, T. B. (2007). Stability and specificity of meaning in life and life satisfaction over one year. *Journal of Happiness Studies*, *8*(2), 161–179. doi:10.1007/s10902-006-9011-8

Steger, M. F., Oishi, S., & Kashdan, T. B. (2009). Meaning in life across the life span: Levels and correlates of meaning in life from emerging adulthood to older adulthood. *The Journal of Positive Psychology*, *4*(1), 43–52. doi:10.1080/17439760802303127

Steuber, K. R., & Solomon, D. H. (2011). Factors that predict married partners' disclosures about infertility to social network members. *Journal of Applied Communication Research*, *39*(3), 250–270. doi:10.1080/00909882.2011.585401

Su, T. J., Chen, H. F., Chen, H. F., Yang, Y. S., & Hung, Y. T. (2006). Factors related to meaning of life in Taiwanese women treated with in vitro fertilization. *Journal of the Formosan Medical Association*, *105*(5), 404–413.

Van den Broeck, U., D'Hooghe, T., Enzlin, P., & Demyttenaere, K. (2010). Predictors of psychological distress in patients starting IVF treatment: Infertility-specific versus general psychological characteristics. *Human Reproduction*, *25*(6), 1471–1480. doi:10.1093/humrep/deq030

Vassard, D., Lund, R., Pinborg, A., Boivin, J., & Schmidt, L. (2012). The impact of social relations among men and women in fertility treatment on the decision to terminate treatment. *Human Reproduction*, *27*(12), 3502–3512. doi:10.1093/humrep/des353

Ying, L. Y., Wu, L. H., & Loke, A. Y. (2015). Gender differences in experiences with and adjustments to infertility: A literature review. *International Journal of Nursing Studies*, *52*(10), 1640–1652. doi:10.1016/j.ijnurstu.2015.05.004

Perinatal Maternal Stress and Susceptibility to Infectious Diseases in Later Childhood: An Early Life Programming Perspective

Irena Stepanikova, Elizabeth Baker, Gabriela Oates, Sanjeev Acharya, Jalal Uddin, Vojtech Thon, Jan Svancara, and Lubomir Kukla

ABSTRACT

There is evidence of transmission of stress-related dysregulation from parents to offspring during early developmental stages, leading to adverse health outcomes. This study investigates whether perinatal stress is linked to the risk of infectious diseases in children aged 7–11 years. We hypothesize that stress exposure during pregnancy and the first 6 months after birth independently predict common infectious diseases. Data are obtained from ELSPAC-CZ, a prospective birth cohort. Maternal stress, operationalized as the number of life events, is examined for pregnancy and the first 6 months postpartum. Children's diseases include eye infection, ear infection, bronchitis/lung infection, laryngitis, strep throat, cold sores, and flu/flu-like infection. More prenatal and postnatal life events are both independently linked to a higher number of infectious diseases between the ages of 7–11 years. The effect is larger for postnatal vs. prenatal events, and the effect of prenatal events is attenuated after maternal health in pregnancy is controlled. The results suggest that perinatal stress is linked to susceptibility to infectious diseases in school-age children. Interventions to address stress in pregnant and postpartum women may benefit long-term children's health.

Since Walter Cannon (1935) and Hans Selye (1956) first described the stress response in living organisms, scholars have sought to understand the health consequences of exposure to stressors. The early formulations of the stress theory focused on the effects of stress on the exposed individual. However, stress-related dysregulation is not limited to the person directly experiencing the stressor. Individuals who have a relationship with the exposed person can develop adverse outcomes as well. The parent–child relationship is a prime example. Psychologists, educators, sociologists, and pediatricians have long noted developmental, emotional, and behavioral problems among children from families that face difficult life situations, such as death, divorce, homelessness, forced migration, persecution, war, or terror. Traditionally, these adverse effects have been attributed to children's vicarious experience of parental stress, disruptions of routines in the child's daily life, and changes in parental behavior, such as less time spent with the child, less consistent parenting, and greater use of punitive discipline.

The interest in biological pathways linking parental stress to offspring health is relatively recent and is rooted in animal models (Blaze & Roth, 2015). Increased levels of stress hormones among pregnant laboratory animals predict a variety of long-term adverse outcomes for the neurobiological and behavioral development of the offspring (Weinstock, 2005). Stress-related changes in the parental organism can be directly transmitted to offspring through several mechanisms, most notably gametes and gestational uterine environment (Bowers & Yehuda, 2016). This biological transmission, known as "intergenerational transmission of stress" (Bowers & Yehuda, 2016), is distinct from social and behavioral pathways through which parental stress influences children, for instance through parental behavior toward the child.

In humans, prenatal stress as a risk factor for adverse health outcomes has been documented in a study of mothers exposed to Tutsi genocide during pregnancy (Perroud et al., 2014). Children of these mothers later showed a dysfunction of the hypothalamic-pituitary-adrenal (HPA) axis. Prenatal anxiety, a proxy for stress during pregnancy, has been linked to brain development in newborns (Qiu et al., 2015) and in children aged 6–9 years (Buss, Davis, Muftuler, Head, & Sandman, 2010), as well as to externalizing problems, ADHD symptoms, and anxiety in children age 8 and 9 years (Van den Bergh & Marcoen, 2004). In another study, higher cortisol levels in amniotic fluid, indicating higher levels of maternal stress, predicted lower cognitive ability among 17-month-old children (Bergman, Sarkar, Glover, & O'Connor, 2010). Arguably, stress exposure during pregnancy can predispose the developing fetus to a variety of pathophysiological processes through its dysregulating influence on neurodevelopment, glucocorticoid levels (Cottrell & Seckl, 2009), HPA axis function (Glover, O'Connor, & O'Donnell, 2010), and maternal–placental–fetal immune processes (Entringer, Buss, & Wadhwa, 2010). Epigenetic changes, namely methylation in the promoter of *NR3C1*, have also been reported (Mulligan, D'Errico, Stees, & Hughes, 2012; Radtke et al., 2011).

Intergenerational transmission implies that the effects of parental stress during the early developmental stages are long-lasting, extending well beyond infancy and early childhood. In fact, several studies find that individuals exposed to stress in utero show various adverse outcomes as adults. Yehuda, Bell, Bierer, & Schmeidler (2008), for instance, compared children of Holocaust survivors and demographically similar Jewish controls. Adult children of Holocaust survivors had higher lifetime risk of depression, anxiety, and post-traumatic stress disorder. Similarly, women exposed to the stress of starvation during the Dutch famine of 1945–1946 had children who reported poorer mental health and lower overall quality of life in mid-adulthood as compared to counterparts (Stein, Pierik, Verrips, Susser, & Lumey, 2009). Higher risk of insulin resistance and shorter telomere length were found in young adults whose mothers had experienced adverse life events during pregnancy (Entringer et al., 2008, 2011).

The goal of the present study is to examine whether psychosocial stress during the perinatal period, defined as pregnancy and the first 6 months after birth, influences the risk of common infectious diseases in later childhood. We focus on infectious diseases because they remain a major source of children's morbidity and mortality worldwide (Bryce, Boschi-Pinto, Shibuya, Black, & WHO Child Health Epidemiology Reference Group, 2005; Liu et al. 2012), constitute a large part of pediatric ambulatory visits (Poehling et al., 2013; West, 2002), and are associated with considerable economic and social costs (Fairbrother et al., 2010; Fendrick, Monto, Nightengale, & Sarnes, 2003). Annual cost burden of emergency care for influenza in young children in the US, for instance, is estimated at $44–$163 million (Fairbrother et al., 2010). Additionally, the social and economic implications of common infections in children include absences from school and extracurricular activities as well as missed work and lost income for caregivers. A parent caring for a child with the flu misses 73 work hours on average, with incurred costs of $1,456 (Fama & Dwibedi, 2015). Common pediatric infections rarely require hospitalization, but complications do occur, such as hearing loss with otitis media (Hunter, Margolis, & Giebink, 1994) or acute rheumatic fever with Group A *Streptococcus* infection (Felsenstein et al., 2014). Importantly, some infections, such as those affecting airways and ear, are often treated with broad-spectrum antibiotics, sometimes without laboratory testing to specify the type of infectious agent. This practice raises concerns about overprescribing and antibiotic resistance, both pressing issues from the perspective of current population health (Fossum, Lindbaek, Gjelstad, Dalen, & Kvaerner, 2013; Pichichero, 1999).

Increased vulnerability to infections among individuals experiencing stressful life situations has been long noted. In 1964, empirical evidence was obtained using retrospective observational data from patients with pulmonary tuberculosis (Rahe, Meyer, Smith, Kjaer, & Holmes, 1964). In this patient population, life changes requiring major social readjustment peaked during the 2-year period preceding the onset of tuberculosis. Experimental evidence corroborating the stress-infection linkage was presented several decades later in a study by Cohen, Tyrrel, & Smith (1991). Healthy adult volunteers were exposed to nasal drops with five strains of respiratory viruses and subsequently quarantined. Subjects who reported higher levels of stress were more likely to develop a respiratory infection after exposure. Along with findings from several other studies (Glaser et al., 1992; Kiecolt-Glaser, Glaser, Gravenstein, Malarkey, & Sheridan, 1996), this evidence suggests that under stress, the adult immune system is less effective in warding off infections.

In a few studies, the idea of stress as a factor in immune functioning was extended to the population of pregnant women and children. O'Connor et al. (2013) demonstrated that prenatal maternal depression and anxiety, proxies for stress, were associated with reduced adaptive immunity among 6-month-old infants as indicated by humoral immune response to Hepatitis B vaccine. In another study, innate and adaptive immune responses were assessed using cord blood. Altered immune responses were observed for newborns whose mothers scored higher on a composite stress measure including financial hardship, difficult life circumstances, and community violence during pregnancy (Wright et al., 2010). A study that compared newborns delivered by forceps or vacuum, a proxy for stress, to newborns delivered in a less stressful manner, found that forceps/vacuum deliveries had higher lymphocyte subset counts in cord blood (Duijts et al., 2008).

Regarding maternal stress and common infectious diseases in childhood, two observational studies of infants suggest that prenatal stress relates to an increased risk. In a large Norwegian birth cohort, stressful life events during pregnancy were associated with the frequency and variety of infectious diseases during the first year of life (Henriksen & Thuen, 2015). A smaller study of 174 Dutch mothers with normal pregnancies and term deliveries linked pregnancy-specific anxiety and stress during the last trimester to infant illness and antibiotic treatment (Beijers, Jansen, Riksen-Walraven, & de Weerth, 2010). Evidence concerning children beyond their first year of life is limited to a large Danish birth-cohort study, which documents that the number of hospitalizations for infectious diseases among children aged 0–14 years increases when the mothers report having experienced death of a spouse, death of an older child, or divorce during pregnancy or up to 3 years before conception (Nielsen, Hansen, Simonsen, & Hviid, 2011).

While the reviewed evidence suggests greater susceptibility to infectious diseases among children exposed to stress in utero, it also leaves unanswered several important questions. First, little is known about the impact of maternal stress on the risk of infectious diseases after infancy. The Danish cohort study discussed earlier examined children up to 14 years of age, but it was limited to relatively rare life events, e.g., death in the family or divorce. While such events are intensely stressful, they are a thin slice of the wide range of events that may induce stress during pregnancy, including serious stressors such as crime and violence, loss of a job or home, serious illness in the family, pregnancy complications, and concerns about the health of the unborn child. Additionally, less severe but more common events, such as marital discord or other types of interpersonal conflict, financial difficulties, and problems at work, can take a toll on the health of the pregnant woman and her child, especially when these problems are chronic and difficult to resolve. In this study, we address the gap in evidence by evaluating a wide range of potentially stressful life events to achieve a more comprehensive understanding of perinatal maternal stress and its effect on the child.

Second, prior research has focused chiefly on prenatal stress as a factor in childhood infections, to the exclusion of postnatal stress. The postpartum period is inherently stressful for many women. Mothers experience profound physical and hormonal changes, sleep deprivation, challenges with lactation and infant feeding, role strain caused by competing demands of infant care and other social roles, fatigue, and, commonly, anxiety and affective problems that can escalate into postpartum depression. At the same time, the infant body and mind are developing rapidly during these earliest phases of life. The development of multiple physiological systems at this stage is characterized by great plasticity and sensitivity to influences from the environment, and the effects of dysregulation at this stage are long-lasting. Disturbances in early parenting among mothers with postpartum depression, for instance, have been linked to increased waking cortisol levels among 13-year-old adolescents (Murray, Halligan, Goodyer, & Herbert, 2010). Immune development is no exception. Evidence indicates that immune programming starts in utero and continues during early life (Renz, Brandtzaeg, & Hornef, 2011). If a fetus or infant is exposed to stress, early immune programing can become dysregulated (Bilbo & Schwarz, 2009) and increase the risk of developing infectious diseases in later life, when the child is more exposed to infections through interaction with children and adults outside of the family.

Building on these arguments, we propose the following hypotheses:

> H1: Prenatal stress is positively related to common infectious diseases in school-aged children.

H2: Postnatal stress is positively related to common infectious diseases in school-aged children.

To test these hypotheses, we leverage longitudinal birth-cohort data from the Czech Republic. We focus on stressful life events during pregnancy and the first 6 months postpartum and relate them to common infectious diseases among children aged 7-11 years.

Data

Data were obtained from the European Longitudinal Study of Pregnancy and Childhood, the Czech Republic (ELSPAC-CZ). ELSPAC-CZ, modeled after the Avon Longitudinal Study of Pregnancy and Childhood (ALSPAC) (Golding, Pembrey, & Jones, 2001), is part of the European Longitudinal Study of Pregnancy and Childhood (ELSPAC) (ELSPAC, 1989), a multisite prospective birth-cohort study initiated by the World Health Organization to identify factors that affect the health of pregnant women and children in Europe. ELSPAC-CZ was approved by the Scientific Committee of Masaryk University. The detailed description of the design, methodology, and characteristics of ELSPAC-CZ cohort are provided by Piler et al. (2016). The goal of ELSPAC-CZ was to reach the entire population of births in Brno and Znojmo districts of the Czech Republic between March 1, 1991 and June 30, 1992. Inclusion criteria were expected date of delivery within the targeted period and a permanent address in one of the study districts. Pregnant women were recruited in collaboration with local obstetricians and gynecologists. All participants provided written informed consent. Pen-and-paper questionnaires were distributed in mid-pregnancy to 7,262 women. The response rate was 71% ($N = 5{,}167$).

This analysis uses maternal questionnaires completed at baseline, 6 months after delivery, and around the child's 11th birthday, when mothers reported the occurrence of common infectious diseases in the focal child between the ages of 7 and 11 years. At age 11, 2,609 mothers responded to the survey. We also use data collected from maternal medical charts to determine pregnancy characteristics and birth outcomes. Three hundred fifty-six questionnaires (7%) were excluded because of missing identification. To avoid potential bias due to shared genetic and family characteristics, twins ($N = 80$) were also excluded. Of the remaining sample, roughly 9% of cases had missing data on the analytic variables. Missing data were accounted for by using multiple imputations (MI). To determine if the data were missing at random, a dichotomous indicator representing missing values on any of the predictor values was created and used in the full model to predict the main dependent and independent variables. The effect of this variable was not statistically significant, suggesting that data were missing at random, and MI were deemed appropriate (Acock, 2005). Ten MI datasets were created and analyzed using Stata 14.2 with a sample size of 2,075. Results for the imputed and non-imputed data were similar.

Measures

Perinatal Stress: Prenatal and Postnatal Life Events

To asses stress, we used life events questionnaire based on the work of Barnett, Hanna, & Parker (1983) and Honnor, Zubrick, & Stanley (1994) and previously used in the

ALSPAC study. The questionnaire has been used extensively in prior research (Araya et al., 2009; Dewey, Fleming, Golding, & ALSPAC Study Team, 1998; Dorrington et al., 2014; Dunn et al., 1998; Enoch, Steer, Newman, Gibson, & Goldman, 2010; Hibbeln et al., 2007; Rai et al., 2012; Sullivan, Rai, Golding, Zammit, & Steer, 2013). Examples of items include "You moved house," "Your house or car was burgled," and "Your partner had trouble with law." The instrument had two forms: prenatal and postpartum. The prenatal questionnaire asked women about events that had taken place since the beginning of their pregnancy, while the postpartum questionnaire asked about events that had occurred between delivery and 6 months postpartum. Both common and rare life events were included, ranging from job loss and relationship conflicts to divorce and death in the family. In addition, each questionnaire version included events specific to that particular life period. For instance, pregnant women were asked whether during the pregnancy they had bleeding and thought they might miscarry, while at 6 months, participants were asked whether they had become pregnant since delivery. Questionnaires included 41 different types of potentially stressful events for each period (see Appendix for the complete list of events). We calculated a total number of events reported for each period. The life event indicators had a right-skewed distribution (prenatal events, skewness = .51; postnatal events, skeweness = 7.77). To account for skewness and potential nonlinearity between life events and infections, both indicators were dichotomized based on, roughly, the median response. For both observed periods, having three or more life events is referred to henceforth as high stress while having two or fewer events is referred to as low stress.

Infectious Diseases in Mid-childhood

Around the child's 11th birthday, mothers were presented with a list of diseases and asked to report whether their child had each disease between the ages of 7 and 11 years. We focus on seven diseases that are likely to have an infectious origin (henceforth referred to as "infectious diseases"): eye infection, ear infection, bronchitis/lung infection, laryngitis, strep throat, cold sores on the lips, and flu/flu-like infection. Responses for each were yes = 1 vs. no = 0. The total number of reported infectious diseases was calculated (range: 0–7), reflecting the *variety* of infectious diseases rather than the frequency of illness, which was not measured. Counts of infectious diseases reported by parents have been used as a measure of child illness in prior research (Duijts, Jaddoe, Hofman, & Moll, 2010; Duijts et al., 2008). Polychoric inter-item correlations ranged from .14 to .39. The Kuder–Richardson coefficient (Kuder & Richardson, 1937) was .46. This score is low because the variable represents a count and does not measure a unidimensional underlying concept. Because of a skewed distribution (skewness = .51), the variable was log-transformed in multivariate models.

Control variables

Demographic characteristics used as covariates in all models included maternal age at delivery, maternal marital status (married vs. not married), and years of education as an indicator of socioeconomic status. To proxy parity, we used pregnant women's reports of whether they had children and coded nulliparous women as 1 and others as 0. These factors were measured by self-report in mid-pregnancy.

Among other control variables, maternal *health behaviors* with known implications for child health were included. These were smoking and alcohol use during pregnancy (Fergusson, Woodward, & Horwood, 1998; Latino-Martel et al., 2010) and breastfeeding (Eidelman et al., 2012). Pregnant women reported whether they had smoked during the past 9 months and consumed alcohol during the past month (yes = 1 vs. no = 0). Breastfeeding was measured at 6 months, with mothers reporting whether they currently breastfed the child (yes = 1 vs. no = 0). Self-reports of *maternal health during pregnancy* were included as well. Women were asked whether during pregnancy they experienced nausea/vomiting, diarrhea, flu/flu-like symptoms, urinary tract infection, and yeast infection (each coded yes = 1 vs. no = 0). In addition, they reported self-rated health on a scale from 1 ("always poor") to 5 ("excellent"). Finally, *characteristics of the delivery* were collected from maternal medical charts. A dichotomous (0/1) indicator for intrapartum complications was coded as "1" when any of the following were noted in the chart: edema, fever, prolonged first-stage labor, prolonged second-stage labor, arrested labor, alterations in fetal heartbeat, meconium in amniotic fluid, uterine abruption, eclampsia, umbilical cord prolapse, umbilical cord coiled around neck, and obstructed labor. Low/very low birth weight (LBW) was defined as <2,500 g. The mode of delivery was coded as cesarean section vs. other. The child's sex (female vs. male) was recorded as well.

Analysis

Analyses were conducted using Stata statistical software, version 14.2. After obtaining descriptive and bivariate statistics, we estimated a series of nested multivariate linear regression models using as an outcome variable the index totaling infectious diseases in mid-childhood. All models with the count variable of total number of types of infections used Huber-White estimators (Huber, 1967; White, 1980), which relax the assumptions of normality and homoscedasticity, yielding robust estimates in the presence of non-normal distributions and heteroscedasticity. All models controlled for demographic factors measured at baseline (mid-pregnancy), in accordance with guidelines by the European Medicines Agency (2013) regarding the adjustment for baseline covariates. Model 1 used prenatal life events as the main explanatory variable. Model 2 added postnatal life events. Model 3 added factors related to maternal health, including maternal health behaviors, health during pregnancy, and characteristics of the delivery. As the next step, a series of logistic regression models predicting the likelihood of each individual infectious disease were estimated using a similar modeling strategy as described above.

Based on the results from the nested multivariate regression models, additional analyses were conducted to examine mediation using inverse odds ratio weighting (IORW; Nguyen et al., 2015; Tchetgen Tchetgen, 2013). This technique has several advantages including being agnostic to the presence or absence of treatment-mediator interactions, allowing for multiple mediators and covariates, and being able to accommodate semi-parametric and nonparametric models. This technique condenses the relationship

Table 1. Characteristics of the Sample.

	Mean/percentage	*SE*
Perinatal stress		
≥3 prenatal life events	50.3%	.01
≥3 postnatal life events	48.1%	.01
Health status in pregnancy		
Self-rated health	3.84	.02
Nausea/vomiting	78.5%	.01
Diarrhea	13.1%	.01
Urinary tract infection	2.8%	.00
Flu/flu-like infection	25.1%	.01
Yeast infection	6.4%	.01
Health behaviors		
Alcohol consumption in pregnancy	6.1%	.01
Smoking in pregnancy	18.2%	.01
Breastfeeding at 6 months	27.0%	.01
Delivery characteristics		
Intrapartum complications	25.1%	.01
Cesarean section	7.7%	.01
Low birth weight (<2,500 g)	2.9%	.004
Male child	50.1%	.01
Demographic background		
Education (years)	12.3	.06
Married	89.5%	.01
Age at delivery (years)	25.9	.10
Nulliparous	50.9%	.01

Notes. Estimates of mean or percentage are shown.
SE = standard error. Source: European Longitudinal Study of Pregnancy and Childhood-Czech Republic (ELSPAC-CZ). Estimates are obtained using multiple imputations with chained equations (MICE); $N = 2{,}075$.

between the treatment and the mediator(s) into a weight, which is the inverse of the conditional odds predicting the treatment as a function of the mediator(s) and covariates. This weight is then applied to the regression model predicting the outcome as a function of the treatment and covariates. This is the natural direct effect. The total effect is estimated by predicting the outcome as a function of the treatment and the covariates, and the natural indirect effect is estimated as the difference between these two. Since the method to calculate the bootstrapped standard errors for these paths does not accommodate multiple imputations, we performed mediation analyses on non-imputed data.

Results

At baseline, most participants were married (89.5%), with a mean of 12.3 years of education (Table 1). The mean age at delivery was 25.9 years. Approximately half (51.0%) of the women were nulliparous. One or more intrapartum complications were present in 25.1% of cases. Fewer than one in ten deliveries were caesarian sections (7.7%) and roughly one in fifty had LBW (2.9%). Reports of alcohol consumption during pregnancy were rare (6.1%), but nearly every fifth pregnant woman reported smoking (18.2%). Despite overall good self-reported health in pregnancy (mean = 3.84 on a 1–5 scale), most women reported nausea/vomiting (78.5%), and a quarter reported having had the flu/flu-like infection (25.1%). Reports of diarrhea, urinary tract infection, and yeast infection during pregnancy were less common (13.1%; 2.8%, and 6.4%, respectively). As far as perinatal life stress, women reported on average 3.01 prenatal and 2.24 postnatal

Table 2. Infectious Diseases for Children Age 7–11 years, Maternal Report.

	Percentage/mean	*SE*
Type of infectious disease		
Eye infection	9.2%	.01
Ear infection	12.4%	.01
Flu/flu-like infection	75.8%	.01
Cold sores	22.2%	.01
Laryngitis	20.7%	.01
Bronchitis/lung infection	27.4%	.01
Strep throat	53.1%	.01
Total of types of infectious diseases	1.9	.01

Notes. Estimates of mean or percentage are shown.
SE = standard error. Source: European Longitudinal Study of Pregnancy and Childhood-Czech Republic (ELSPAC-CZ). Estimates are obtained using multiple imputations with chained equations (MICE); $N = 2{,}075$.

life events; because of the skewness, these variables were dichotomized for multivariate analysis at roughly the median as three or more vs. two or fewer.

The most commonly reported infectious disease in children ages 7–11 years was flu/flu-like infection (75.8%), followed by strep throat (53.1%), bronchitis/lung infection (27.4%), cold sores (22.2%), and laryngitis (20.7%) (Table 2). Eye and ear infections were rarer (9.2% and 12.4%, respectively). Mothers reported an average of 1.9 types of infectious diseases experienced by their children between ages 7 and 11.

Consistent with our hypotheses, the results of multivariate models indicate that perinatal life events predict the total types of infectious diseases in mid-childhood (Table 3). In Model 1, which includes only prenatal life events and demographic covariates, the unstandardized coefficient for the effect of high prenatal stress on the log of total types of infectious diseases is .11 (95% CI: .07, .16, $p < .001$), indicating that the expected total types of infectious diseases are 11% higher for those who experienced three or more prenatal life events as compared to two or fewer events. The magnitude of the statistical effect for prenatal life events is virtually un-attenuated ($b = .11$, 95% CI: .05, .14, $p < .001$) after including postnatal life events in Model 2 and the effect of prenatal life events remains statistically significant, supporting Hypothesis 1. Model 3 includes the measures of maternal health status, health behaviors, and delivery characteristics and further reduces the association between prenatal stress and infectious diseases though this association retains significance ($b = .06$, 95% CI: .04, .13, $p = .008$), suggesting only partial mediation.

Consistent with Hypothesis 2, life events during the 6 months after delivery predict the total types of infectious diseases during mid-childhood, with three or more life events postpartum increasing the expected total types of infections by 9% ($b = .09$, 95% CI: .05, .14, $p < .001$). The effect of postnatal events remains virtually un-attenuated after adjusting for maternal health factors in Model 3 ($b = .08$, 95% CI: .04, .13, $p = .001$). At the same time, several self-reported health problems in pregnancy emerge as significant predictors of child's infectious diseases. The largest effect is observed for maternal flu/flu-like infection ($b = .12$, 95% CI: .06, .17, $p < .001$), followed by diarrhea ($b = .11$, 95% CI: .04, .18, $p = .002$), and nausea/vomiting ($b = .09$, 95% CI: .03, .15, $p = .002$). Prenatal smoking and alcohol use are not related to the child's infectious diseases but more educated mothers have children with fewer types of infectious diseases

Table 3. Linear Regression Models of the Total of Types of Infectious Diseases for Children Age 7-11 years.

	Model 1			Model 2			Model 3		
	b	[95% CI]	*p*	*b*	[95% CI]	*p*	*b*	[95% CI]	*p*
Perinatal stress									
≥3 prenatal life events	**.11**	[.07, .16]	<.001	**.10**	[.05, .14]	<.001	**.06**	[.02, .11]	.008
≥3 postnatal life events				**.09**	[.05, .14]	<.001	**.08**	[.04, .13]	.001
Demographic background									
Education, years	**−.01**	[−.02, −.00]	.036	**−.01**	[−.02, −.00]	.035	**−.01**	[−.02, −.00]	.027
Married	−.02	[−.09, .05]	.603	−.01	[−.09, .06]	.704	−.02	[−.10, .05]	.456
Age at delivery, years	−.00	[−.01, .01]	.676	−.00	[−.01, .00]	.836	.00	[−.001, .01]	.920
Nulliparous	−.02	[−.07, .02]	.344	−.01	[−.06, .04]	.617	−.01	[−.06, .04]	.724
Health status in pregnancy									
Self-rated health							−.02	[−.05, .01]	.141
Nausea/vomiting							**.09**	[.03, .15]	.002
Diarrhea							**.11**	[.04, .18]	.002
Urinary tract infection							.05	[−.08, .18]	.411
Flu/flu-like infection							**.12**	[.06, .17]	<.001
Yeast infection							.04	[−.06, .15]	.408
Health behaviors									
Alcohol use in pregnancy							−.03	[−.14, .07]	.565
Smoking in pregnancy							.03	[−.03, .09]	.304
Breastfeeding at 6 months							**.06**	[.004, .11]	.035
Delivery characteristics									
Intrapartum complications							.02	[−.03, .07]	.493
Cesarean section							−.05	[−.13, .03]	.223
Low birth weight (<2,500 g)							.05	[−.08, .17]	.455
Male child							.00	[−.04, .05]	.859

Notes. b = unstandardized regression coefficient; CI = confidence interval.
p values are for two-tailed tests. Bold indicates $p < .05$. The total of types of infectious diseases was log-transformed for multivariate models. Source: European Longitudinal Study of Pregnancy and Childhood-Czech Republic (ELSPAC-CZ). Estimates are obtained using multiple imputations with chained equations (MICE); $N = 2{,}075$.

($b = -.01$, 95% CI: −.02, −.001, $p = .027$) and breastfeeding at 6 months is positively associated with infectious diseases ($b = .06$, 95% CI: .004, .11, $p = .035$).

Next, we investigated the role of perinatal stress for each individual infectious disease (Table 4). Without taking into account postnatal life events and maternal health, prenatal life events are linked to increased odds of all examined diseases, with the exception of the ear infections and laryngitis (Model 1). For other diseases, Hypothesis 1 is supported. Compared to those with two or fewer events, the odds of bronchitis/lung infection are 47% higher for those with three or more events (95% CI: 1.22, 1.77, $p < .001$). Increases in the odds associated with higher prenatal stress are 37% for eye infection (95% CI: 1.09, 1.71, $p = .007$), 36% for flu/flu-like infection (95% CI: 1.10, 1.68, $p = .005$), 37% for strep throat (95% CI: 1.15, 1.64, $p = .001$), and 26% for cold sores (95% CI: 1.04, 1.53, $p = .016$). After including postnatal life events in Model 2, Hypothesis 1 remains supported for strep throat (OR = 1.30, 95% CI: 1.08, 1.56, $p = .005$), bronchitis/lung infection (OR = 1.37, 95% CI: 1.13, 1.65, $p = .001$), eye infections (OR = 1.26, 95% CI: 1.00, 1.59, $p = .048$), and the flu (OR = 1.31, 95% CI: 1.05, 1.63, $p = .014$). At the same time, postnatal life events *independently* predict increased odds of eye infections (OR: 1.49, 95% CI: 1.17, 1.89, $p = .001$), bronchitis/lung infection (OR: 1.42, 95% CI: 1.17, 1.72, $p < .001$), cold sores (OR: 1.42, 95% CI: 1.16, 1.73, $p = .001$), laryngitis (OR: 1.36, 95% CI: 1.11, 1.67, $p = .003$), ear infections (OR: 1.33, 95% CI 1.06, 1.68, $p = .016$), and strep throat (OR: 1.31, 95% CI: 1.09, 1.58, $p = .004$), providing support for Hypothesis 2. After accounting for postnatal events, prenatal life events

Table 4. Odds Ratios from Logistic Regression Models of Infectious Diseases for Children Age 7–11 years.

	Bronchitis/ lung infection		Ear infection		Strep throat		Cold sores		Eye infection		Flu/flu-like infection		Laryngitis	
	OR	[95% CI]	OR	[95% CI]	OR	[95% CI]	OR	[95% CI]	OR	[95% CI]	OR	[95% CI]	OR	[95% CI]
Model 1[a]														
≥3 prenatal life events	**1.47**	[1.22, 1.77] $p<.001$	1.10	[.88, 1.37] $p=.395$	**1.37**	[1.15, 1.64] $p=.001$	**1.26**	[1.04, 1.53] $p=.016$	**1.37**	[1.09, 1.71] $p=.007$	**1.36**	[1.10, 1.68] $p=.005$	1.19	[.98, 1.44] $p=.081$
Model 2[a]														
≥3 prenatal life events	**1.37**	[1.13, 1.65] $p=.001$	1.04	[.83, 1.30] $p=.746$	**1.30**	[1.08, 1.56] $p=.005$	1.18	[.97, 1.43] $p=.102$	**1.26**	[1.00, 1.59] $p=.048$	**1.31**	[1.05, 1.63] $p=.014$	1.11	[.91, 1.35] $p=.301$
≥3 postnatal life events	**1.42**	[1.17, 1.72] $p<.001$	**1.33**	[1.06, 1.68] $p=.016$	**1.31**	[1.09, 1.58] $p=.004$	**1.42**	[1.16, 1.73] $p=.001$	**1.49**	[1.17, 1.89] $p=.001$	1.19	[.96, 1.49] $p=.120$	**1.36**	[1.11, 1.67] $p=.003$
Model 3[b]														
≥3 prenatal life events	**1.26**	[1.03, 1.53] $p=.023$	.97	[.77, 1.22] $p=.771$	**1.25**	[1.03, 1.50] $p=.021$	1.09	[.89, 1.34] $p=.388$	1.16	[.91, 1.48] $p=.212$	1.24	[.99, 1.54] $p=.059$	1.01	[.82, 1.24] $p=.930$
≥3 postnatal life events	**1.36**	[1.12, 1.66] $p=.002$	**1.28**	[1.01, 1.63] $p=.039$	**1.26**	[1.04, 1.52] $p=.017$	**1.39**	[1.13, 1.71] $p=.002$	**1.42**	[1.11, 1.80] $p=.005$	1.18	[.94, 1.48] $p=.149$	**1.29**	[1.05, 1.59] $p=.016$

Notes. OR = odds ratio; CI = confidence interval.
[a]Controlling for demographic background.
[b]Controlling for demographic background indicators, health status in pregnancy, health behaviors, and delivery characteristics. p values are for two-tailed tests. Bold indicates $p < .05$.
Source: European Longitudinal Study of Pregnancy and Childhood-Czech Republic (ELSPAC-CZ). Estimates are obtained using multiple imputations with chained equations (MICE). $N = 2,075$.

are no longer a significant predictor for cold sores and flu. When maternal health status and health behaviors are controlled (Model 3), prenatal life events are no longer a significant predictor for eye infections, while postnatal life events remain a significant predictor for laryngitis (OR: 1.29, 95% CI: 1.05, 1.59, $p = .016$), strep throat (OR: 1.26, 95% CI: 1.04, 1.52, $p = .017$), cold sores (OR: 1.39, 95% CI: 1.13, 1.71, $p = .002$), ear infections (OR: 1.28, 95% CI: 1.01, 1.63, $p = .039$), eye infections (OR: 1.42, 95% CI: 1.11, 1.80, $p = .005$), and bronchitis/lung infection (OR: 1.36, 95% CI: 1.12, 1.66, $p = .002$).

To formally test mediation for models in which the effect of prenatal events did not retain statistical significance, we used IORW approach to calculate the indirect paths. The results indicate a significant indirect path through postnatal life events in the model for cold sores ($b_{\text{indirect}} = .14$, 95% CI: .05, .22, $p = .001$). Additionally, the indirect path through maternal health and health behaviors was found for eye infection ($b_{\text{indirect}} = .45$, 95% CI: .17, .73, $p = .001$). In contrast, in the model of flu/flu-like infection, indirect pathways through postnatal life events or through maternal health and health behaviors were not significantly different from zero.

Discussion and Limitations

Using longitudinal data from a large Czech birth cohort, this study examined the role of perinatal stress for subsequent infectious diseases in school-aged children. It focused specifically on stressful life events experienced by mothers during pregnancy and the first 6 months of the child's life. Results indicate that both prenatal and postnatal stress predict infectious diseases in mid-childhood, but the postnatal life events have stronger and more consistent effects across types of common pediatric infections.

Prenatal and postnatal stress, as indicated by life events, is correlated, suggesting that women who experience a high number of life events in pregnancy are also likely to experience an increased number of life events postpartum. When measures of postnatal stress are included among predictors of infectious diseases in mid-childhood, the contribution of prenatal stress is attenuated, though both prenatal and postnatal stress remain important independent predictors of child health. This is a noteworthy finding. Prior research has examined prenatal stress, documenting that stress-related changes in hormonal and immune functioning during pregnancy have long-term effects on the child's immune system, neuro-cognitive development, and overall health status (Ruiz & Avant, 2005). Less is known about the ways in which susceptibility to infections in later life is influenced by maternal stress exposure during the first months of the child's life, although maternal postpartum depression and anxiety have been linked to adverse health outcomes for the child (O'hara & McCabe, 2013). A separate body of literature argues that early life adversity, such as abuse, neglect, or trauma, predicts higher morbidity and mortality in later life (Johnson, Riley, Granger, & Riis, 2013). Pediatricians caution about "toxic stress," defined as "the extreme, frequent, or extended activation of the stress response, without the buffering presence of a supportive adult" (Johnson et al., 2013). Our findings extend further these lines of research by showing that stress from a wide range of maternal life events, not just severely traumatic events, influence the child's long-term health.

This study was not intended to specify the biological mechanisms linking maternal stress to infections in offspring. Nevertheless, the results are provocative and raise questions about the implications of maternal exposure to stressors for the child's immune development and functioning. They resonate with emerging evidence that stress during sensitive periods of early life leads to immune dysregulation, manifested, for instance, as an excessive inflammatory response to microbial stimulation and resistance to inhibitory mechanisms that lower inflammation (Miller, Chen, & Parker, 2011). Alterations of the quality of microbiome passed from mother to infant during vaginal delivery and through breastmilk may also play a role. Microbial colonization of the gut is known to play a critical role in the development of systems and functions implicated in immune response, including neuro-immune system, HPA axis, and metabolic status (Jašarević, Howerton, Howard, & Bale, 2015; Kozyrskyj & Sloboda, 2016).

We did examine maternal health status in pregnancy and characteristics of the delivery as potential mechanisms linking perinatal stress to child infections and found that the total number of types of infectious diseases in school-aged children increased with several self-reported maternal health problems during pregnancy, namely maternal flu/flu-like infection, nausea/vomiting, and diarrhea. Notably, all these maternal health problems could potentially indicate infection. In fact, we found that the association between prenatal life events and infectious diseases is attenuated once we account for maternal health. These findings suggest that prenatal stress increases the risk of health problems during pregnancy, which may later lead to the child's greater susceptibility to infections. We are not aware of studies relating infections among pregnant women to infections in school-aged children specifically, prior research has suggested other types of adverse effects for infections during pregnancy, including congenital malformations and neuro-cognitive dysfunctions potentially leading to schizophrenia and autism in the child (Patterson, 2009). Maternal infections, however, represent only one potential mechanism through which prenatal stress impacts child's health, as only partial mediation occurred in our study. Further studies using objective markers of maternal and child infection, as opposed to self-reports, along with measures of other mediators are needed to better understand these patterns.

Limitations of the study must be noted. First, the cohort consisted predominantly of young women (mean age = 25.2 years) with low rates of cesarean delivery (8.1%). These characteristics are consistent with the demographic composition of the Czech population at the time of the study (Bobak, 2000; Srp & Velebil, 1999) but may limit the generalizability to older mothers and complicated pregnancies. Second, children's infectious diseases were measured by maternal reports. During the pilot phase of the study, mothers' understanding of medical terms used in the survey (e.g., "flu," "bronchitis") was queried. No problems with understanding were noted. Nonetheless, it cannot be assumed that all mothers had the knowledge needed to accurately diagnose medical conditions. Some degree of under-reporting (a child had a disease, but the mother did not report it), over-reporting (a child did not have a disease but the mother reported it), and misreporting (a child had one type of disease but the mother reported it as another) cannot be ruled out. Still, maternal reports of child's health status are routinely used in health surveys (McCormick, Athreya, Bernbaum, & Charney, 1988), as they are cost-effective and have an important advantage in capturing a broad range of health conditions. Unlike data from chart reviews, mothers' reports include conditions for which medical care may not have been sought. This is especially true for minor infections, such as herpes simplex or laryngitis, which commonly resolve without medical attention. Having data, albeit reported by mothers, on whether the child has had these diseases is important for a comprehensive picture of the child's overall health.

It must be reiterated that mothers reported whether their children had each type of disease during the specified age period but did not indicate the number of times each disease occurred. This means that we cannot identify children experiencing repeated infections of a single type (e.g., repeated bronchitis). Furthermore, we have no data on disease severity and course, which could be important from the perspective of the child's immune functioning and health more broadly. Finally, for stress, participants reported types of life events experienced during pregnancy and postpartum periods but not the number of times each event occurred. Some types of life events, such as divorce, marriage, or death of a spouse, are unlikely to occur more than once during the reporting periods (9 months prenatal and 6 months postnatal). Other events, such as job loss, change of employment, or residential move, could have taken place repeatedly, potentially increasing the overall stress level for the mother. Finally, despite the fact that our survey covered a wider range of life events compared to most prior studies, the list was not exhaustive and some participants could have experienced stress because of unmeasured situations.

Despite these limitations, study findings suggest that maternal stress during the first 6 months postpartum distinctly increases the child's risk of common infections in mid-childhood. Notably, the role of postnatal stress as a risk factor for infectious diseases in mid-childhood is independent of prenatal stress for some types of infections. These findings suggest that postnatal stress plays a role in the link between prenatal stress and child health. Stress during pregnancy may influence the child's long-term health via different processes. The first one involves mother-fetal-placental interaction, as suggested by the independent pathways from prenatal stress to the risk of infectious disease in our data. The second process, discussed briefly earlier, involves increased risk of health problems, e.g., infections, in stressed pregnant women. The third process may be rooted in the relationship between life events in pregnancy and life events after delivery. It is reminiscent of Pearlin's (1989) concept of stress proliferation. Pearlin (1989) argues that stressors have a tendency to generate a cascade of further stressful events in a person's life. An adverse life event can give rise to ongoing strains in various areas of life even after the acute stressor is no longer longer present. This eventually can lead to more adverse events, increasing the overall stress exposure for the individual. For instance, a pregnant woman going through a divorce (stressor 1) may face financial difficulties because of the loss of spousal income (stressor 2) and may accept living arrangements that involve crowding (stressor 3) and noise (stressor 4) or may seek unsanitary housing (stressor 5) in a neighborhood that exposes her to crime and violence (stressor 6). In this example, the original stressor of divorce led to a proliferation of stresses and strains, which persisted long after the divorce was no longer an acute stressor.

Conclusions

Given our findings, interventions to address stress during pregnancy and postpartum should be considered because of their long-term benefits for the health of the child.

Stress-related counseling is available to some pregnant women and to women who had a distressing delivery experience (Gamble & Creedy, 2004). Women diagnosed with postpartum depression often receive psychological counseling as a part of therapy. Yet for many women, stress assessment and psychological interventions are not available although pregnancy and the time after delivery are stressful periods of great adjustment for the woman and her family. Opportunities for perinatal stress screening should be identified, and interventions should be implemented to help a wide range of women receive services that can offset the harmful effects of maternal stress on the health of their children.

Acknowledgments

The authors of this study wish to thank the participating families as well as the gynecologists, pediatricians, school heads and class teachers who took part in the project. Our thanks also go to Lubomír Kukla, Ph.D., ELSPAC national coordinator 1990–2012, and the entire ELSPAC team. The authors of this study (i.e., not the ELSPAC Scientific Council) are responsible for the content of this publication.

Ethics approval and consent to participate

ELSPAC-CZ was approved by the Scientific Committee of Masaryk University. All participants provided written informed consent.

Funding

This study was funded by the Ministry of Education, Youth and Sports of the Czech Republic and European Structural and Investment Funds (CETOCOEN PLUS project: CZ.02.1.01/0.0/0.0/15_003/0000469 and the RECETOX research infrastructure: LM2015051 and CZ.02.1.01/0.0/0.0/16_013/0001761).

Data availability statement

ELSPAC-CZ data can be requested via http://www.elspac.cz/index-en.php?pg=professionals.

References

Acock, A. C. (2005). Working with missing values. Journal of Marriage and Family, 67(4), 1012–1028. doi:10.1111/j.1741-3737.2005.00191.x

Araya, R., Hu, X., Heron, J., Enoch, M. A., Evans, J., Lewis, G., … ., Goldman, D. (2009). Effects of stressful life events, maternal depression and 5-HTTLPR genotype on emotional symptoms in pre-adolescent children. American Journal of Medical Genetics Part B: Neuropsychiatric Genetics, 150(5), 670–682. doi:10.1002/ajmg.b.30888

Barnett, B. E., Hanna, B., & Parker, G. (1983). Life event scales for obstetric groups. Journal of Psychosomatic Research, 27(4), 313–320. doi:10.1016/0022-3999(83)90054-5

Beijers, R., Jansen, J., Riksen-Walraven, M., & de Weerth, C. (2010). Maternal prenatal anxiety and stress predict infant illnesses and health complaints. Pediatrics, 126(2), e401–e409. doi:10.1542/peds.2009-3226

Bergman, K., Sarkar, P., Glover, V., & O'Connor, T. G. (2010). Maternal prenatal cortisol and infant cognitive development: Moderation by infant–mother attachment. Biological Psychiatry, 67(11), 1026–1032. doi:10.1016/j.biopsych.2010.01.002

Bilbo, S. D., & Schwarz, J. M. (2009). Early-life programming of later-life brain and behavior: A critical role for the immune system. Frontiers in Behavioral Neuroscience, 14(3), 14. doi:10.3389/neuro.08.014.2009

Blaze, J., & Roth, T. L. (2015). Evidence from clinical and animal model studies of the long-term and transgenerational impact of stress on DNA methylation. Seminars in Cell & Developmental Biology, 43, 76–84. doi:10.1016/j.semcdb.2015.04.004

Bobak, M. (2000). Outdoor air pollution, low birth weight, and prematurity. Environmental Health Perspectives, 108(2), 173–176.

Bowers, M. E., & Yehuda, R. (2016). Intergenerational transmission of stress in humans. Neuropsychopharmacology, 41(1), 232–244. doi:10.1038/npp.2015.247

Bryce, J., Boschi-Pinto, C., Shibuya, K., Black, R. E., & WHO Child Health Epidemiology Reference Group (2005). WHO estimates of the causes of death in children. Lancet, 365(9465), 1147–1152. doi:10.1016/S0140-6736(05)71877-8

Buss, C., Davis, E. P., Muftuler, L. T., Head, K., & Sandman, C. A. (2010). High pregnancy anxiety during mid-gestation is associated with decreased gray matter density in 6–9-year-old children. Psychoneuroendocrinology, 35(1), 141–153. doi:10.1016/j.psyneuen.2009.07.010

Cannon, W. B. (1935). Stress and strains of homeostasis. American Journal of Medical Science, 189(1), 13–14.

Cohen, S., Tyrrell, D. A., & Smith, A. P. (1991). Psychological stress and susceptibility to the common cold. The New England Journal of Medicine, 325(9), 606–612. doi:10.1056/NEJM199108293250903

Cottrell, E. C., & Seckl, J. R. (2009). Prenatal stress, glucocorticoids and the programming of adult disease. Frontiers in Behavioral Neuroscience, 3, 19. doi:10.3389/neuro.08.019.2009

Dewey, C., Fleming, P., & Golding, J. & ALSPAC Study Team (1998). Does the supine sleeping position have any adverse effects on the child? II. Development in the first 18 months. Pediatrics, 101(1), e5–e5. doi:10.1542/peds.101.1.e5

Dorrington, S., Zammit, S., Asher, L., Evans, J., Heron, J., & Lewis, G. (2014). Perinatal maternal life events and psychotic experiences in children at twelve years in a birth cohort study. Schizophrenia Research, 152(1), 158–163. doi:10.1016/j.schres.2013.11.006

Duijts, L., Bakker, J., L. E., Labout, J. A., Jaddoe, V. W., Hofman, A., Steegers, E. A., … Moll, H. A. (2008). Perinatal stress influences lymphocyte subset counts in neonates. The generation R study. Pediatric Research, 63(3), 292–298. doi:10.1203/PDR.0b013e318163a29f

Duijts, L., Jaddoe, V., W., Hofman, A., & Moll, H. A. (2010). Prolonged and exclusive breastfeeding reduces the risk of infectious diseases in infancy. Pediatrics, 126(1), e18–e25. doi:10.1542/peds.2008-3256

Duijts, L., Jaddoe, V., W., Hofman, A., Steegers, E., A., Mackenbach, J., P., D., Jongste, J., C., & Moll, H. A. (2008). Maternal smoking in prenatal and early postnatal life and the risk of respiratory tract infections in infancy. The Generation R study. European Journal of Epidemiology, 23(8), 547–555. doi:10.1007/s10654-008-9264-0

Dunn, J., Deater-Deckard, K., Pickering, K., O'Connor, T., G., & Golding, J. & ALSPAC Study Team (1998). Children's adjustment and prosocial behaviour in step-, single-parent, and non-stepfamily settings: Findings from a community study. Journal of Child Psychology and Psychiatry, 39(8), 1083–1095. doi:10.1111/1469-7610.00413

Eidelman, A. I., Schanler, R. J., Johnston, M., Landers, S., Noble, L., Szucs, K. & Viehmann, (2012). Breastfeeding and the use of human milk. Pediatrics, 129(3), e827–e841. doi:10.1542/peds.2011-3552

ELSPAC. (1989). European Longitudinal Study of Pregnancy and Childhood (ELSPAC). Paediatric and Perinatal Epidemiology, 3(4), 460–469. doi:10.1111/j.1365-3016.1989.tb00533.x

Enoch, M., A., Steer, C., D., Newman, T., K., Gibson, N., & Goldman, D. (2010). Early life stress, MAOA, and gene-environment interactions predict behavioral disinhibition in children. Genes, Brain and Behavior, 9(1), 65–74. doi:10.1111/j.1601-183X.2009.00535.x

Entringer, S., Buss, C., & Wadhwa, P. D. (2010). Prenatal stress and developmental programming of human health and disease risk: Concepts and integration of empirical findings. Current Opinion in Endocrinology, Diabetes, and Obesity, 17(6), 507. doi:10.1097/MED.0b013e3283405921

Entringer, S., Epel, E. S., Kumsta, R., Lin, J., Hellhammer, D. H., Blackburn, E. H., … Wadhwa, P. D. (2011). Stress exposure in intrauterine life is associated with shorter telomere length in young adulthood. Proceedings of the National Academy of Sciences, 108(33), E513–E518. doi:10.1073/pnas.1107759108

Entringer, S., Wüst, S., Kumsta, R., Layes, I. M., Nelson, E. L., Hellhammer, D. H., & Wadhwa, P. D. (2008). Prenatal psychosocial stress exposure is associated with insulin resistance in young adults. American Journal of Obstetrics and Gynecology, 199(5), 498.e1. doi:10.1016/j.ajog.2008.03.006

European Medicines Agency. (2013). Guideline on adjustment for baseline covariates in clinical trials EMA/CHMP/295050/2013. http://www.ema.europa.eu/docs/en_GB/document_library/Scientific_guideline/2015/03/WC500184923.pdf

Fairbrother, G., Cassedy, A., Ortega-Sanchez, I. R., Szilagyi, P. G., Edwards, K. M., Molinari, N.-A., … Staat, M. A. (2010). High costs of influenza: Direct medical costs of influenza disease in young children. Vaccine, 28(31), 4913–4919. doi:10.1016/j.vaccine.2010.05.036

Fama, J. P., & Dwibedi, N. (2015). Effect of pediatric influenza on caregivers' burden: A literature review. Journal of Human Behavior in the Social Environment, 25(6), 522–529. doi:10.1080/10911359.2014.884963

Felsenstein, S., Faddoul, D., Sposto, R., Batoon, K., Polanco, C. M., & Bard, J. D. (2014). Molecular and clinical diagnosis of group A streptococcal pharyngitis in children. Journal of Clinical Microbiology, 52(11), 3884–3889. doi:10.1128/JCM.01489-14

Fendrick, A. M., Monto, A. S., Nightengale, B., & Sarnes, M. (2003). The economic burden of non–influenza-related viral respiratory tract infection in the United States. Archives of Internal Medicine, 163(4), 487–494. doi:10.1001/archinte.163.4.487

Fergusson, D. M., Woodward, L. J., & Horwood, L. J. (1998). Maternal smoking during pregnancy and psychiatric adjustment in late adolescence. Archives of General Psychiatry, 55(8), 721–727. doi:10.1001/archpsyc.55.8.721

Fossum, G. H., Lindbaek, M., Gjelstad, S., Dalen, I., & Kvaerner, K. J. (2013). Are children carrying the burden of broad-spectrum antibiotics in general practice? Prescription pattern for paediatric outpatients with respiratory tract infections in Norway. BMJ Open, 3(1), e002285. doi:10.1136/bmjopen-2012-002285

Gamble, J., & Creedy, D. (2004). Content and processes of postpartum counseling after a distressing birth experience: A review. Birth (Berkeley, CA), 31(3), 213–218. doi:10.1111/j.0730-7659.2004.00307.x

Glaser, R., Kiecolt-Glaser, J. K., Bonneau, R. H., Malarkey, W., Kennedy, S., & Hughes, J. (1992). Stress-induced modulation of the immune response to recombinant hepatitis B vaccine. Psychosomatic Medicine, 54(1), 22–29. doi:10.1097/00006842-199201000-00005

Glover, V., O'Connor, T. G., & O'Donnell, K. (2010). Prenatal stress and the programming of the HPA axis. Neuroscience: Biobehavioural Review, 35(1), 17–22. doi:10.1016/j.neubiorev.2009.11.008

Golding, J., Pembrey, M., & Jones, R. (2001). ALSPAC—The Avon longitudinal study of parents and children. I. Study methodology. Paediatric and Perinatal Epidemiology, 15(1), 74–87. doi:10.1046/j.1365-3016.2001.00325.x

Henriksen, R. E., & Thuen, F. (2015). Marital quality and stress in pregnancy predict the risk of infectious disease in the offspring: the Norwegian mother and child cohort study. PloS One, 10(9), e0137304. doi:10.1371/journal.pone.0137304

Hibbeln, J., R., Davis, J., M., Steer, C., Emmett, P., Rogers, I., Williams, C., & Golding, J. (2007). Maternal seafood consumption in pregnancy and neurodevelopmental outcomes in childhood (ALSPAC study): An observational cohort study. Lancet, 369(9561), 578–585. doi:10.1016/S0140-6736(07)60277-3

Honnor, M. J., Zubrick, S. R., & Stanley, F. J. (1994). The role of life events in different categories of preterm birth in a group of women with previous poor pregnancy outcome. European Journal of Epidemiology, 10(2), 181–188. doi:10.1007/BF01730368

Huber, P. J. (1967, June). The behavior of maximum likelihood estimates under nonstandard conditions. In Proceedings of the fifth berkeley symposium on mathematical statistics and probability (Vol. 1;, pp. 221–233). Berkeley and Los Angeles: University of California Press.

Hunter, L. L., Margolis, R. H., & Giebink, G. S. (1994). Identification of hearing loss in children with otitis media. Annals of Otology, Rhinology and Laryngology, 103(5_Suppl), 59–61. doi:10.1177/00034894941030S516

Jašarević, E., Howerton, C. L., Howard, C. D., & Bale, T. L. (2015). Alterations in the vaginal microbiome by maternal stress are associated with metabolic reprogramming of the offspring gut and brain. Endocrinology, 156(9), 3265–3276. doi:10.1210/en.2015-1177

Johnson, S. B., Riley, A. W., Granger, D. A., & Riis, J. (2013). The science of early life toxic stress for pediatric practice and advocacy. Pediatrics, 131(2), 319–327. doi:10.1542/peds.2012-0469

Kiecolt-Glaser, J. K., Glaser, R., Gravenstein, S., Malarkey, W. B., & Sheridan, J. (1996). Chronic stress alters the immune response to influenza virus vaccine in older adults. Proceedings of the National Academy of Sciences, 93(7), 3043–3047. doi:10.1073/pnas.93.7.3043

Kozyrskyj, A. L., & Sloboda, D. M. (2016). Perinatal programming of gut microbiota and immunity. Journal of Developmental Origins of Health and Disease, 7(01), 2–4. doi:10.1017/S2040174415007916

Kuder, G. F., & Richardson, M. W. (1937). The theory of the estimation of test reliability. Psychometrika, 2(3), 151–160. doi:10.1007/BF02288391

Latino-Martel, P., Chan, D. S., Druesne-Pecollo, N., Barrandon, E., Hercberg, S., & Norat, T. (2010). Maternal alcohol consumption during pregnancy and risk of childhood leukemia: Systematic review and meta-analysis. Cancer Epidemiology and Prevention Biomarkers, 19(5), 1238–1260. doi:10.1158/1055-9965.EPI-09-1110

Liu, L., Johnson, H. L., Cousens, S., Perin, J., Scott, S., Lawn, J. E., ... Black, R. E. (2012). Global, regional, and national causes of child mortality: an updated systematic analysis for 2010 with time trends since 2000. Lancet, 379(9832), 2151–2161. doi:10.1016/S0140-6736(12)60560-1

McCormick, M. C., Athreya, B. H., Bernbaum, J. C., & Charney, E. B. (1988). Preliminary observations on maternal rating of health of children: data from three subspecialty clinics. Journal of Clinical Epidemiology, 41(4), 323–329. doi:10.1016/0895-4356(88)90139-4

Miller, G. E., Chen, E., & Parker, K. J. (2011). Psychological stress in childhood and susceptibility to the chronic diseases of aging: Moving toward a model of behavioral and biological mechanisms. Psychological Bulletin, 137(6), 959–997. doi:10.1037/a0024768

Mulligan, C., D'Errico, N., Stees, J., & Hughes, D. (2012). Methylation changes at NR3C1 in newborns associate with maternal prenatal stress exposure and newborn birth weight. Epigenetics, 7(8), 853–857. doi:10.4161/epi.21180

Murray, L., Halligan, S. L., Goodyer, I., & Herbert, J. (2010). Disturbances in early parenting of depressed mothers and cortisol secretion in offspring: a preliminary study. Journal of Affective Disorders, 122(3), 218–223. doi:10.1016/j.jad.2009.06.034

Nguyen, Q. C., Osypuk, T. L., Schmidt, N. M., Glymour, M. M., & Tchetgen Tchetgen, E. J. (2015). Practical guidance for conducting mediation analysis with multiple mediators using inverse odds ratio weighting. American Journal of Epidemiology, 181(5), 349–356. doi:10.1093/aje/kwu278

Nielsen, N. M., Hansen, A. V., Simonsen, J., & Hviid, A. (2011). Prenatal stress and risk of infectious diseases in offspring. American Journal of Epidemiology, 173(9), 990–997. doi:10.1093/aje/kwq492

O'Connor, T. G., Winter, M. A., Hunn, J., Carnahan, J., Pressman, E. K., Glover, V., ... Caserta, M. T. (2013). Prenatal maternal anxiety predicts reduced adaptive immunity in infants. Brain, Behavior, and Immunity, 32, 21–28. doi:10.1016/j.bbi.2013.02.002

O'hara, M. W., & McCabe, J. E. (2013). Postpartum depression: current status and future directions. Annual Review of Clinical Psychology, 9(1), 379–407. doi:10.1146/annurev-clinpsy-050212-185612

Patterson, P. H. (2009). Immune involvement in schizophrenia and autism: etiology, pathology and animal models. Behavioural Brain Research, 204(2), 313–321. doi:10.1016/j.bbr.2008.12.016

Pearlin, L. I. (1989). The sociological study of stress. Journal of Health and Social Behavior, 30(3), 241–256. doi:10.2307/2136956

Perroud, N., Rutembesa, E., Paoloni-Giacobino, A., Mutabaruka, J., Mutesa, L., Stenz, L., ... Karege, F. (2014). The Tutsi genocide and transgenerational transmission of maternal stress: Epigenetics and biology of the HPA axis. The World Journal of Biological Psychiatry, 15(4), 334–345. doi:10.3109/15622975.2013.866693

Pichichero, M. E. (1999). Understanding antibiotic overuse for respiratory tract infections in children. Pediatrics, 104(6), 1384–1388. doi:10.1542/peds.104.6.1384

Piler, P., Kandrnal, V., Kukla, L., Andrýsková, L., Švancara, J., Jarkovský, J., ..., Klánová, J. (2016). Cohort profile: The European Longitudinal Study of Pregnancy and Childhood (ELSPAC) in the Czech Republic. International Journal of Epidemiology, 46(5), 1379–1379. doi:10.1093/ije/dyw091

Poehling, K. A., Edwards, K. M., Griffin, M. R., Szilagyi, P. G., Staat, M. A., Iwane, M. K., ... Bridges, C. B. (2013). The burden of influenza in young children, 2004–2009. Pediatrics, 131(2), 207–216. doi:10.1542/peds.2012-1255

Qiu, A., Tuan, T. A., Ong, M. L., Li, Y., Chen, H., Rifkin-Graboi, A., ... Meaney, M. J. (2015). COMT haplotypes modulate associations of antenatal maternal anxiety and neonatal cortical morphology. American Journal of Psychiatry, 172(2), 163–172. doi:10.1176/appi.ajp.2014.14030313

Radtke, K. M., Ruf, M., Gunter, H. M., Dohrmann, K., Schauer, M., Meyer, A., & Elbert, T. (2011). Transgenerational impact of intimate partner violence on methylation in the promoter of the glucocorticoid receptor. Translational Psychiatry, 1(7), e21. doi:10.1038/tp.2011.21

Rahe, R. H., Meyer, M., Smith, M., Kjaer, G., & Holmes, T. H. (1964). Social stress and illness onset. Journal of Psychosomatic Research, 8(1), 35–44. doi:10.1016/0022-3999(64)90020-0

Rai, D., Golding, J., Magnusson, C., Steer, C., Lewis, G., & Dalman, C. (2012). Prenatal and early life exposure to stressful life events and risk of autism spectrum disorders: Population-based studies in Sweden and England. PloS One, 7(6), e38893. doi:10.1371/journal.pone.0038893

Renz, H., Brandtzaeg, P., & Hornef, M. (2012). The impact of perinatal immune development on mucosal homeostasis and chronic inflammation. Nature Reviews Immunology, 12(1), 9. nri3112. doi:10.1038/nri3112

Ruiz, R. J., & Avant, K. C. (2005). Effects of maternal prenatal stress on infant outcomes: A synthesis of the literature. Advances in Nursing Science, 28(4), 345–355. doi:10.1097/00012272-200510000-00006

Selye, H. (1956). The stress of life. New York: McGraw-Hill.

Srp, B., & Velebil, P. (1999). Proportion of caesarean sections and main causes of maternal mortality during 1978-1997 in the Czech Republic. Ceska Gynekologie, 64(4), 219–223.

Stein, A. D., Pierik, F. H., Verrips, G. H. W., Susser, E. S., & Lumey, L. H. (2009). Maternal exposure to the Dutch famine before conception and during pregnancy: Quality of life and depressive symptoms in adult offspring. Epidemiology (Cambridge, MA), 20(6), 909–915. doi: 10.1097/EDE.0b013e3181b5f227

Sullivan, S., Rai, D., Golding, J., Zammit, S., & Steer, C. (2013). The association between autism spectrum disorder and psychotic experiences in the Avon longitudinal study of parents and children (ALSPAC) birth cohort. Journal of the American Academy of Child and Adolescent Psychiatry, 52(8), 806–814. doi:10.1016/j.jaac.2013.05.010

Tchetgen Tchetgen, E. J. (2013). Inverse odds ratio-weighted estimation for causal mediation analysis. Statistics in Medicine, 32(26), 4567–4580. doi:10.1002/sim.5864

Van Buuren, S., Boshuizen, H. C., & Knook, D. L. (1999). Multiple imputation of missing blood pressure covariates in survival analysis. Statistics in Medicine, 18(6), 681–694. doi:10.1002/(SICI)1097-0258(19990330)18:6%3C681::AID-SIM71%3E3.0.CO;2-R

Van den Bergh, B. R., & Marcoen, A. (2004). High antenatal maternal anxiety is related to ADHD symptoms, externalizing problems, and anxiety in 8-and 9-year-olds. Child Development, 75(4), 1085–1097. doi:10.1111/j.1467-8624.2004.00727.x

Weinstock, M. (2005). The potential influence of maternal stress hormones on development and mental health of the offspring. Brain, Behavior, and Immunity, 19(4), 296–308. doi:10.1016/j.bbi.2004.09.006

West, J. V. (2002). Acute upper airway infections: Childhood respiratory infections. British Medical Bulletin, 61(1), 215–230. doi:10.1093/bmb/61.1.215

White, H. (1980). A heteroskedasticity-consistent covariance matrix estimator and a direct test for heteroskedasticity. Econometrica: Journal of the Econometric Society, 48(4), 817–838.

Wright, R. J., Visness, C. M., Calatroni, A., Grayson, M. H., Gold, D. R., Sandel, M. T., ... Gern, J. E. (2010). Prenatal maternal stress and cord blood innate and adaptive cytokine responses in an inner-city cohort. American Journal of Respiratory and Critical Care Medicine, 182(1), 25–33. doi:10.1164/rccm.200904-0637OC

Yehuda, R., Bell, A., Bierer, L. M., & Schmeidler, J. (2008). Maternal, not paternal, PTSD is related to increased risk for PTSD in offspring of Holocaust survivors. Journal of Psychiatric Research, 42(13), 1104–1111. doi:10.1016/j.jpsychires.2008.01.002

Appendix

Table A1. Life Events During Pregnancy Assessed in ELSPAC-CZ.

1. Your partner died
2. One of your children died
3. A friend or relative died
4. One of your children was ill
5. Your partner was ill
6. A friend or relative was ill
7. You were admitted to hospital
8. You were in trouble with the law
9. You were divorced
10. You found that your partner didn't want your child
11. You were very ill
12. Your partner lost his job
13. Your partner had problems at work
14. You had problems at work
15. You lost your job
16. Your partner went away
17. Your partner was in trouble with the law
18. You and your partner separated
19. Your income was reduced
20. You argued with your partner
21. You had arguments with your family or friends
22. You moved house
23. Your partner hurt you physically
24. You became homeless
25. You had a major financial problem
26. You got married
27. Your partner hurt your children physically
28. You attempted suicide
29. You were convicted of an offence
30. You were bleeding and thought you might miscarry
31. You started a new job
32. You had a test to see if your baby was abnormal
33. You had a result on a test that suggested your baby might not be normal
34. You were told that you were going to have twins
35. You heard that something that had happened might be harmful to the baby
36. You tried to have an abortion
37. You took an examination
38. Your partner was emotionally cruel to you
39. Your partner was emotionally cruel to your children
40. Your house or car was burgled
41. You had an accident

Table A2. Life Events During the First 6 Months Postpartum Assessed in ELSPAC-CZ.

1. Your partner died
2. One of your children died
3. A friend or relative died
4. One of your children was ill
5. Your partner was ill
6. A friend or relative was ill
7. You were admitted to hospital
8. You were in trouble with the law
9. You were divorced
10. You found that your partner didn't want your child
11. You were very ill
12. Your partner lost his job
13. Your partner had problems at work
14. You had problems at work
15. You lost your job
16. Your partner went away
17. Your partner was in trouble with the law
18. You and your partner separated
19. Your income was reduced
20. You argued with your partner
21. You had arguments with your family or friends
22. You moved house
23. Your partner hurt you physically
24. You became homeless
25. You had a major financial problem
26. You got married
27. Your partner hurt your children physically
28. You hurt your children physically
29. You attempted suicide
30. You were convicted of an offence
31. You became pregnant
32. You started a new job
33. You returned to work
34. You had a miscarriage
35. You had an abortion
36. You took an examination
37. Your partner was emotionally cruel to you
38. Your partner was emotionally cruel to your children
39. You were emotionally cruel to your children
40. Your house or car was burgled
41. You had an accident

Moderating Effects of Prevention-Focus on the Paths from Two Insecure Attachment Dimensions to Depression

Dong-Gwi Lee, Jae Joon Park, Byeong Hoon Bae and Hyun-Woo Lim

ABSTRACT
The present study investigated the moderating effects of prevention-focus on the paths from the dimensions of insecure attachment (attachment avoidance and attachment anxiety) to depression. Two hundred twenty eight Korean college students completed the Experience in Close Relationship – Revised Scale; the Regulatory Focus Strategies Scale; and the Center for Epidemiologic Studies Depression Scale. Results revealed a significant moderating effect for prevention-focus on the path from attachment avoidance to depression, but not on the path from attachment anxiety to depression. They further suggest that different interventions are needed for different combinations of persons' insecure attachment dimensions and levels of prevention-focus. Counseling implications and suggestions for future research are discussed.

Introduction

Depression is one of the most prevalent mental disorders in South Korea, costing over 7 to 10 trillion Korean Won (63 to 85 billion US Dollars) per year over the five-year period from 2007 to 2011 (Lee, Baek, Yoon, & Kim, 2013). The number of patients diagnosed with depression has increased steadily, a 12% increase in 2015 from 2011. Moreover, the lifetime prevalence of depression diagnosis has increased progressively from 4.0% in 2001 through 5.6% in 2006, to 6.7% in 2011 (Korean Health Insurance Review & Assessment Service, 2015). This high rate is also cross-cultural; according to Blazer, Kessler, McGonagle, and Swartz (1994), 17.1% of the US population (15–54 years of age) suffer from depressive disorder at one time or another during their lifetime. Depression is such a common illness that detailed investigation of its manifold causes or precedent variables is pivotal.

Depression is conceptualized as a product of the interaction between dysfunctional cognition and negative interpersonal relationship patterns (Safran, 1990). In this conceptualization, the roots of depression can often be found in insecure attachment with childhood caretakers (Whisman & McGarvey, 1995). In fact, several empirical studies on the relationship between attachment and depression in adults have suggested that insecure attachment is a significant precedent variable to predict depression (Besser & Priel, 2003; Gnilka, Ashby, & Noble, 2013; Jinyao et al., 2012; Pietromonaco & Barrett, 1997; Robert, Gotlib, & Kassel,

1996). In particular, a history of insecure attachment, along with self-criticism and dependence, is found to significantly predict depression (Besser & Priel, 2003). Compared to those who have secure attachment, individuals who have insecure attachment are more prone to depression (Myhr, Sookman, & Pinard, 2004; Reis & Grenyer, 2004; Robert et al., 1996).

According to Bowlby's (1973) theory, infants develop an internal working model of attachment based on their relationships with their parents. This internal working model is a cognitive structure containing mental representations for understanding the world, self, and others. Bowlby argued that representations of early attachment patterns become internalized and form the basis for attachment patterns to others in adulthood. Bartholomew and Horowitz (1991) went further to propose four attachment categories (secure, preoccupied, fearful, and dismissing) by splitting the representations of both self and others into positive or negative valence. However, no empirical study has so far determined the exact methods to differentiate the four categories. For this reason, Wei, Mallinckrodt, Russell, and Abraham (2004) argued that attachment is better conceptualized using continuous dimensions, rather than discrete categories.

Insecure attachment fall into two dimensions – attachment avoidance and attachment anxiety (Brennan, Clark, & Shaver, 1998, Cameron, Finnegan, & Morry, 2012). Attachment avoidance is defined as the fear of interpersonal closeness or dependence on others. It can develop when caretakers do not respond to or ignore their children's emotional needs. Attachment anxiety taps the fear of being rejected or abandoned. It can develop when caretakers respond to their children's emotional needs in an inconsistent manner. Those who have insecure attachment are known to resort to two different behavioral strategies (Cassidy, 2000; Ponizovsky & Drannikov, 2013). A deactivating strategy, in which behavior or thought is used to maximize their distance from others and suppress their negative feelings in order to avoid frustration caused by others, is associated with attachment avoidance. In contrast, a hyper-activating strategy, in which behavior or thought is used to maximize their proximity to others and exaggerate their emotional distress in order to elicit others' compassion, reflects attachment anxiety. Wei, Vogel, Ku, and Zakalik (2005) showed that those with high levels of attachment anxiety use emotional reactivity (i.e., a hyper-activating strategy), leading to psychological maladjustment, such as depression, while those who have high levels of attachment avoidance rely on emotional cutoff (i.e., a deactivating strategy), which also results in increased risks of depression.

What remains unexplained in the literature is the inconsistent relationship between attachment avoidance and depression. Some studies found a significant relationship (e.g., Wei, Mallinckrodt, Larson, & Zakalik, 2005) but other studies found no relationship (e.g., Wei, Heppner, Russell, & Young, 2006; Wei, Russell, & Zakalik, 2005), despite the consistent findings about the significant positive association between attachment anxiety and depression (e.g., Simpson & Rholes, 2004; Wei, Mallinckrodt et al., 2005; Wei, Russell et al., 2005). The inconsistent findings regarding the relationship between attachment avoidance and depression indicate that there are different mechanisms involved in the transitions from the two insecure attachment dimensions to depression, and specifically that there exists another variable significantly moderating the path from attachment avoidance to depression.

Our speculation is further supported by a previous study (Wei, Mallinckrodt, Russell, & Abraham, 2004) which examined possible moderating effects of some selected psychological attributes (e.g., maladaptive perfectionism, couple adaptation, etc.) on the links between the two insecure attachment dimensions and depression. Wei et al. (2004) found that maladaptive perfectionism significantly moderates the link from attachment anxiety to depression but not the link from attachment avoidance to depression. The results could be interpreted to suggest that that attachment anxiety, characterized by hyper-activating strategies (e.g., hypervigilance to signs of others' rejection), become more strongly associated with depression when accompanied by excessive worry about others' negative evaluation (i.e., maladaptive perfectionism); in contrast, attachment avoidance, characterized by deactivating strategies (e.g., emotional suppression and defensive distancing), blockades the effect of excessive worry about others' evaluation on the relationship between attachment avoidance and depression. Then the question to be asked is whether there exist other variables that are more sensitive to deactivating strategies which influence the transition from attachment avoidance to depression.

In pursuit of this question, the present study investigated whether "prevention-focus," one of Higgins's (1997) self-regulatory strategies, acts as a moderator of the attachment avoidance–depression relationship. Prevention-focus encompasses the motivation to obtain security, avoid undesired end states, and satisfy one's ought self (Haws, Dholakia, & Bearden, 2010; Higgins, 1997; Klenk, Strauman, & Higgins, 2011). In contrast to promotion-focus which involves advancing success and seeking to attain positive outcomes, prevention-focus reflects behavioral avoidance of threat or failure (Higgins, 1997; Ståhl, van Laar, & Ellemers, 2012). From a motivational perspective, individuals high on prevention-focus scales exhibit a stronger tendency to avoid taking risks to achieve desired outcomes than their counterparts' low said scales (Bryant & Dunford, 2008).

Prevention-focus as a basic motivational principle resembles behavioral manifestations of deactivating strategies to cope with attachment challenges. Given that prevention-focus is positively correlated with perceived stress (Schokker, Links, Luttik, & Hagedoorn, 2010), it could be presumed to be correlated with depression. This may provide a clue to the inconsistent findings regarding the correlations between attachment avoidance and depression found in the literature (e.g., Wei et al., 2006; Wei, Mallinckrodt et al., 2005). It is reasonably inferred that individuals high on prevention-focus would avoid situations likely to include conflict and experience more difficulty in coping with their interpersonal problems. In contrast, those low on prevention-focus are less likely to evade a high-conflict situation and have better chances to resolve their interpersonally problematic situations.

On the other hand, prevention-focus is not likely to act as a moderator of the attachment anxiety–depression relationship as the magnitude of correlation between attachment anxiety and depression is relatively large (e.g., $r = .49$ in Wei et al., 2004). Furthermore, attachment anxiety and a hyper-activating strategy are conceptually unrelated to prevention-focus in that they accompany strong emotional responses than the emotional cut-off and deactivating strategies.

The present study empirically examines the differential moderating effects of prevention-focus on the links between two insecure attachment dimensions (i.e., attachment avoidance and attachment anxiety) and depression in Korean college students. In this study, we aim to contribute to the expanded understanding of the paths from insecure attachment (source variable) to depression (symptom variable) by revealing different mechanisms involved in the two separate insecure attachment dimensions. In addition, we intend to empirically validate the moderating effect of prevention-focus on the attachment avoidance-depression relationship, which provide an explanation for the inconsistent findings regarding attachment avoidance and depression in the previous studies (e.g., Wei et al., 2006; Wei, Mallinckrodt et al., 2005). This study proposes two hypotheses:

Hypothesis 1: Prevention-focus acts as a significant moderator of the attachment avoidance–depression relationship.
Hypothesis 2: Prevention-focus does not act as a significant moderator of the attachment anxiety–depression relationship.

Method

Participants and Procedure

Participants were 228 college students (89 men and 139 women) who enrolled in a psychology course at a private university in Seoul, South Korea. They were comprised of 86 freshman (37.7%), 31 sophomore (13.6%), 54 junior (23.7%), and 58 senior students (25.0%). The average age was 22.27 years ($SD = 2.06$). For this research, IRB review and approval were obtained. We solicited student participation via email, and those who consented to participation completed our online survey using Qualtrics.

Measures

Insecure Attachment Measure

To measure participants' levels of insecure attachment, the Korean version of the Experiences in Close Relationship-Revised (ECR-R) Scale was used. The ECR-R developed by Brennan et al. (1998) was translated and validated in Korean by Kim (2004). The Korean version of the ECR-R consists of two domains including attachment anxiety (18 items, e.g., "I'm afraid that I will lose my partner's love." "I often worry that my partner will not want to stay with me."), attachment avoidance (18 items. e.g., "I prefer not to be too close to romantic partners." "I get uncomfortable when a romantic partner wants to be very close."). The scale includes 10 reverse-coded items and utilizes a Likert format, with response options ranging from 1 (*strongly disagree*) to 5 (*strongly agree*). Higher scores indicate more severe insecure attachment. In Kim (2004), the internal consistencies calculated using Cronbach's alpha statistic (alpha coefficient, hereafter) were .89 for attachment anxiety and .85 for attachment avoidance. In this study, the alpha coefficients for attachment anxiety and attachment avoidance were .77 and .91, respectively.

Prevention-Focus Measure

To measure participants' levels of prevention-focus, the Korean version of the Regulatory Focus Strategies Scale (RFSS) was used. The RFSS developed by Ouschan, Boldero, Kashima, Wakimoto, and Kashima (2007) was translated and validated in Korean by Chun and Lee (2008). The Korean version of the RFSS consists of two domains including promotion focus (8 items) and prevention-focus (8 items. e.g., "To achieve something, it is most important to know all the potential obstacles." "To achieve something, one must be cautious." "To avoid failure, it is important to keep in mind all the potential obstacles that might get in your way."). For the purpose of the study, only the prevention-focus subscale was used. The scale is scored on a 5-point Likert scale (1 = *strongly disagree*, 5 = *strongly agree*) with higher scores indicating higher inclination to use prevention-focus. Chun and Lee (2008) reported the alpha coefficient for prevention-focus to be .79. In this study, the alpha coefficient was calculated as .75.

Depression Measure

To measure participants' levels of depression, we used the Korean version of the Center for Epidemiologic Studies Depression Scale (CES-D). The CES-D developed by Radloff (1977) was translated and validated in Korean by Chon, Choi, and Yang (2001). The scale includes 20 items with a 4-point Likert-type scale (0 = *rarely or none of the time*, 3 = *most or all of the time*) with higher scores indicating higher levels of depressive symptoms (e.g., "I was bothered by things that usually don't bother me." "I did not feel like eating; my appetite was poor."). Chon et al. (2001) reported the alpha coefficient for the CES-D to be .91. In this study, the alpha coefficient was .91.

Data Analysis

To test the moderating effect of prevention-focus on the link between insecure attachment and depression, we used structural equation modeling (SEM), with maximum likelihood estimation, using AMOS 21.0. The use of SEM for examining moderation gives better results than the use of regression analysis. SEM improves the statistical power to detect moderation, by controlling for measurement errors occurring from the low reliability of the interaction term. It further provides a set of overall model-fit indices to determine the adequacy of model fit to the data (Busemeyer & Jones, 1983). In this study, an unconstrained approach was used to estimate the latent interaction among the four factors because the unconstrained approach with imposing no constraints can give an estimate almost identical to that obtained with a fully constrained approach (Marsh, Wen, & Hau, 2004). As the factors (i.e., attachment anxiety, attachment avoidance, prevention-focus, and depression) are unidimensional, item parceling was employed to obtain more precise structural estimates and better model fit. Specifically, we used a domain representative parceling technique (Little, Cunningham, Shahar, & Widaman, 2002) and matched-pair strategy (Jackman, Leite, & Cochrane, 2011) to aggregate item parcels to use as indicators. Mean centering was applied for the indicators of the latent variables to be used for moderator model tests.

Using techniques from Anderson and Gerbing (1988), we examined the fit of the measurement model to the data. Then we tested structural models of interaction among the four measurement factors. Model fit indices used for determining the best fitting model included the Comparative Fit Index (CFI), Tucker–Lewis Index (TLI), Root Mean Square Error of Approximation (RMSEA), and Standardized Root Mean Square Residual (SRMR). The following cut-off values for goodness-of-fit were used: for CFI and TLI .90 or above as an indicator of good fit (Hu & Bentler, 1999); for RMSEA .05 or below good fit and .06–.08 reasonable fit, and below .10 mediocre fit (Browne & Cudeck, 1992); and .06 or below for SRMR good fit (Hu & Bentler, 1999).

Lastly, we inspected how the moderating effect of prevention-focus on the insecure attachment–depression relationship differs by the levels of prevention-focus (high versus low). Given that SEM using AMOS 21.0 does not allow for testing a conditional effect by the levels of a moderator in the relationship between a predictor and a criterion variable (Hayes, 2013a), the process macro (model 1, Hayes, 2013b) in SPSS 21.0 was utilized.

Results

Table 1 provides descriptive statistics and zero-order correlation coefficients for all study variables. Through the item parceling procedure, attachment anxiety had three indicators

Table 1. Descriptive Statistics and Zero-Order Correlation Matrix for the Indicators ($N = 228$).

	1	2	3	4	5	6	7	8	9	10	11	12	13
1. Anxiety 1	—												
2. Anxiety 2	.81***	—											
3. Anxiety 3	.76***	.80***	—										
4. Avoidance 1	.27***	.20**	.39***	—									
5. Avoidance 2	.33***	.28***	.47***	.80***	—								
6. Avoidance 3	.30***	.19**	.37***	.82***	.84***	—							
7. Prevention 1	.32***	.28***	.32***	.23***	.31***	.29***	—						
8. Prevention 2	.25***	.27***	.32***	.22**	.25***	.16*	.60***	—					
9. Prevention 3	.30***	.25***	.38***	.31***	.36***	.34***	.74***	.60***	—				
10. Depression 1	.39***	.29***	.37***	.19**	.18**	.24***	.11	.10	.18**	—			
11. Depression 2	.42***	.39***	.44***	.26***	.29***	.26***	.12	.16*	.16*	.71***	—		
12. Depression 3	.52***	.37***	.44***	.29***	.30***	.31***	.16*	.10	.20**	.70***	.74***	—	
13. Depression 4	.44***	.34***	.45***	.29***	.31***	.35***	.15*	.09	.25***	.74***	.73***	.70***	—
M	3.03	3.75	4.08	3.80	3.87	3.51	4.30	4.74	4.27	1.88	2.17	1.69	1.98
SD	1.03	1.06	1.20	.93	1.02	.98	.95	.87	1.28	.67	.66	.52	.54
Skewness	.22	−.08	−.10	.08	.06	.20	−.39	−.25	−.33	.75	.35	.96	.41
Kurtosis	−.49	−.51	−.46	−.12	−.36	−.25	.57	.03	−.38	−.20	−.33	.56	−.50

*$p < .05$, **$p < .01$, ***$p < .001$.

(anxiety 1, 2, 3); attachment avoidance three indicators (avoidance 1, 2, 3); prevention-focus three indicators (prevention 1, 2, 3); and depression four indicators (depression 1, 2, 3, 4). The indicators all met the normality assumption since no indicator presented skewness and kurtosis value greater than the absolute value of 2 (Tabachnick & Fidell, 2013). The results from the correlation analyses revealed non-significant or weak correlations between the prevention-focus and depression indicators, but significant positive correlations among the remaining indicators.

The results from a confirmatory factor analysis showed that the measurement model was well fitted to the current data [χ^2 (59, $N = 228$) = 157.94, CFI = .96, TLI = .94, RMSEA = .09, & SRMR = .05]. The factor loadings of the indicators ranged from .70 to .92, all above .50, indicating that the indicators adequately represented the latent constructs (Hair, Black, Babin, & Anderson, 2010). Subsequently, testing structural models with the moderation effect of prevention-focus on the relationships among attachment anxiety, attachment avoidance, and depression were performed. The structural model and the path coefficients for the predictor variables are provided by Figure 1 and Table 2.

The results indicated that the moderation model with prevention-focus as a moderator fit the data [χ^2 (137, $N = 228$) = 299.32, CFI = .94, TLI = .92, RMSEA = .07, & SRMR = .05]. In Table 2, the path from the interaction term of avoidance and prevention to depression was significant (b = .21, p < .05), which then supports our Hypothesis 1. On the other hand, the path from the interaction term of anxiety and prevention to depression was not significant (b = −.02, *ns*), which then affirms our Hypothesis 2. In addition, the main effect of attachment anxiety on depression was significant (b = .29, p < .001), indicating that higher degrees of attachment anxiety lead to higher levels of depression. However, the non-significant main effect of prevention focus on depression (b = −.02, *ns*) indicated no direct relationship between those two factors. The estimates for the effect size of moderation of

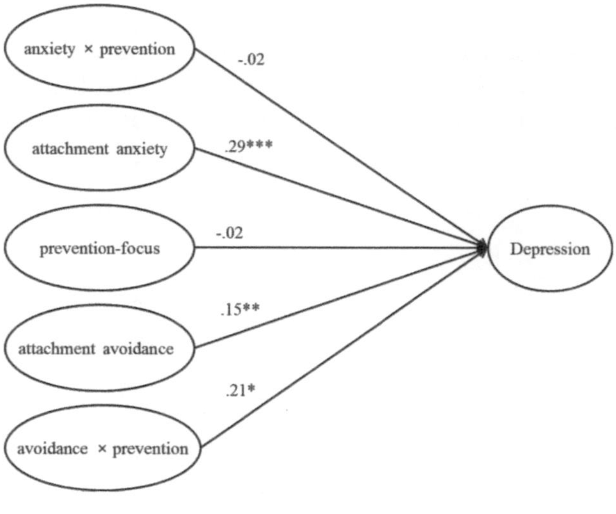

Figure 1. Path Coefficients for the Moderation Effect of Prevention-Focus on the Relationships Between Insecure Attachment and Depression. *Note.* Unstandardized regression coefficients were used for the path coefficients. Covariance estimates for extraneous variables were not provided for the presentation purpose.

Table 2. Path Coefficients for the Moderation Effect of Prevention-Focus on Depression.

Predictors	*b*	*SE*	*β*	*t*
Attachment anxiety	.29	.05	.48	6.34***
Attachment avoidance	.15	.05	.22	3.03**
Prevention-focus	−.02	.05	−.03	−.46
Anxiety × prevention	−.02	.08	−.03	−.26
Avoidance × prevention	.21	.10	.25	2.19*

Note. Beta values for the interaction terms of "anxiety × prevention" and of "avoidance × prevention" were calculated using Wen, Marsh, and Hau (2010) method.
$^{*}p < .05$, $^{**}p < .01$, $^{***}p < .001$.

prevention-focus on the relationship between attachment avoidance and depression (Aiken & West, 1991) was .04, which is a small effect (Cohen, 1992). Given that according to Aguinis, Beaty, Boik, and Pierce (2005), the average effect size in social science research is .01, the effect size of moderation for prevention-focus in this study is considered to be interpretable.

A simple slope test was performed to examine the effect of attachment avoidance on depression at 1 standard deviation (*SD*) above and below the mean value of prevention-focus (Aiken & West, 1991). Hayes's (2013b) process macro (model 1) was used to calculate the values used for the plotting. Figure 2 graphically represents the interaction pattern of prevention-focus on the link from attachment avoidance to depression.

The results demonstrated the robust significant positive effects of attachment avoidance on depression at 1 *SD* above ($b = .12$, $p < .05$) and also at 1 *SD* below ($b = .24$, $p < .001$). Moreover, increased prevention-focus (at 1 *SD* above) has a greater effect on the link from attachment avoidance to depression than does reduced prevention-focus (at 1 *SD* below). This indicates that prevention-focus has exacerbating effects on depression induced from attachment avoidance.

Discussion

The existing literature on attachment has suggested that insecure attachment is related to a range of social and psychological problems including depression (Lopez & Brennan, 2000; Mikulincer & Shaver, 2003). The present study advances the literature by examining differential moderating

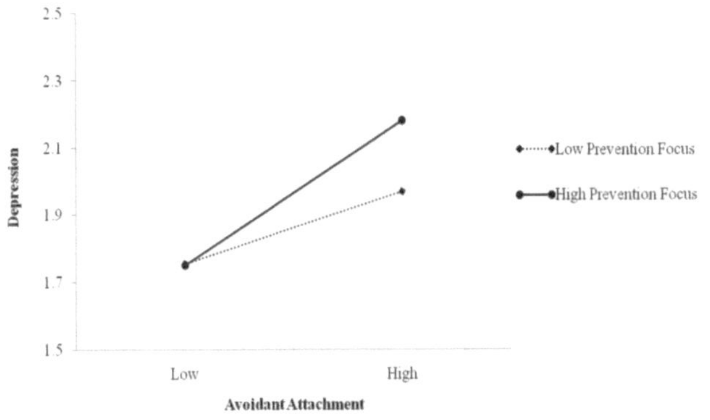

Figure 2. The Moderating Effect of Prevention-Focus on the Relation Between Avoidant Attachment and Depression.

effects of prevention-focus on the paths from insecure attachment's dimensions (attachment avoidance versus attachment anxiety) to depression in particular. The results affirm that prevention-focus acts as a significant moderator for the path from attachment avoidance to depression but not for the path from attachment anxiety to depression. In other words, our results from Korean students indicate that high levels of prevention-focus will intensify the propensity of persons with avoidant attachment to be depressed; avoidant attachment behaviors (emotional suppression and defensive distancing) interact with prevention-focus strategies (avoidance of risk-taking), which could exacerbates their maladaptive interpersonal coping and results in greater propensity toward depression. By contrast, levels of prevention-focus exert no influence on the propensity of persons with the anxious attachment to be depressed.

Our results resonate with the previous findings on attachment and self-regulation (Semin et al., 2005; Wei, Russell et al., 2005). Individuals with high attachment avoidance generally have low trust in others and are less likely to expect emotional support from others (Cann, Norman, Welbourne, & Calhoun, 2008). They tend to be resistant to self-disclosure and interpersonal dependency (DeVito, 2014) and easily motivated to use a deactivating strategy (defensive distancing and emotional cut-off) in pursuing their senses of reassurance (Bryant & Dunford, 2008). Moreover, prevention-focused individuals are inclined to perceive their goals as duties and obligations, and thus experience higher levels of worry and anxiety, than their promotion-focused counterparts (Semin et al., 2005). They act to ensure the absence of negative outcomes that mismatch to desired end-states (Higgins, Roney, Crowe, & Hymes, 1994). Therefore, when individuals with high levels of attachment avoidance have high propensity to use a prevention-focus in coping with their interpersonal conflicts, they are very likely to deny the existence of the problem itself or withdraw from situations they may have to encounter interpersonal problems. This may temporarily fulfill their wish to be self-reliant but increases the possibility of harming relationships, leading to depression in the long run. In addition, our finding of no significant moderating effect of prevention-focus on the path from attachment anxiety to depression seems to support the previous studies where individuals suffering from anxious attachment show excessive fear or anxiety concerning separation from an attachment figure (Park & Lee, 2008; Wallin, 2007). They may use a prevention-focus to gain some reassurance; however, their emotional gains would not affect the progression of attachment anxiety to depressive symptoms.

Overall, the findings of the current study provide useful information for practitioners who work with people who have insecure attachment and depressive symptoms. Counselors may need to examine their clients' levels of prevention-focus, and by alleviating the clients' prevention-focus orientation, help them better cope with loss and fear likely to experience in conflict situations. Thus the intervention for attachment avoidant individuals' depression should include strategies to encourage them to exercise a promotion-focus in their pursuit of interpersonal goals, as alternate strategies to the employment of emotional cut-off and defensive distancing to gain temporal reassurance. On the other hand, when counseling with clients with high levels of attachment anxiety, counselors should be reminded that alleviation of prevention-focus would not be an effective intervention for attachment anxious individuals' depression.

The present study has several limitations. First, regulatory focus theory posits two independent orientations: prevention-focus and promotion-focus. The present study addressed the function of prevention-focus in the transition from insecure attachment to depression only, not that of promotion-focus. We could not include the function of promotion-focus in the analysis, as the data for doing so was not available. Hypothetically, anxious attachment behaviors (hyper-activating strategies) may interact with promotion-focus strategies (advancing success and seeking to attain an attachment figure's approval), which could increase the quality and quantity of interpersonal interactions and consequently prevent depression. Second, in the present study, a cross-sectional research design was used. Thus the relationships reported in this study are correlational; the assessment of cause and effect relationships needs further investigation with a longitudinal research design. Third, the remaining logical possibility is that regulatory focus acts as a mediator, not a moderator, of the insecure attachment–depression relationship.

Despite the aforementioned limitations, the present study has important methodological features that should be highlighted. This study is differentiated from the previous literature, which mostly addressed insecure attachment as a unified variable with few exceptions (e.g., Wei et al., 2006; Wei et al., 2004), in that it examined the subdomains of insecure attachment as two individual variables. Our approach is supported by Park and Lee (2008) which claims that attachment anxiety and attachment avoidance need to be examined separately – the former is associated with mental representations of self and the latter mental representations of others (i.e., positive or negative perceptions of others). In essence, our finding of a significant moderating effect of prevention-focus on the path from attachment anxiety to depression provides an explanation for the inconsistent relationship between attachment avoidance and depression in the literature (e.g., Wei et al., 2006; Wei et al., 2005; Wei, Russell et al., 2005).

References

Aguinis, H., Beaty, J. C., Boik, R. J., & Pierce, C. A. (2005). Effect size and power in assessing moderating effects of categorical variables using multiple regression: A 30-year review. *Journal of Applied Psychology*, *90*(1), 94–107. doi:10.1037/0021-9010.90.1.94

Aiken, L. S., & West, S. G. (1991). *Multiple regression: Testing and interpreting interactions.* Newbury Park, CA: Sage.

Anderson, J. C., & Gerbing, D. W. (1988). Structural equation modeling in practice: A review and recommended two-step approach. *Psychological Bulletin*, *103*(3), 411–423. doi:10.1037/0033-2909.103.3.411

Besser, A., & Priel, B. (2003). A multisource approach to self-critical vulnerability to depression: The moderating role of attachment. *Journal of Personality, 71*(4), 515–555. doi:10.1111/1467-6494.7104002

Bartholomew, K., & Horowitz, L. M. (1991). Attachment styles among young adults: A test of a four-category model. *Journal of Personality and Social Psychology, 61*(2), 226–244. doi:10.1037/0022-3514.61.2.226

Blazer, D. G., Kessler, R. C., McGonagle, K. A., & Swartz, M. S. (1994). The prevalence and distribution of major depression in a national community sample: The national comorbidity survey. *American Journal of Psychiatry, 151*(7), 979–986. doi:10.1176/ajp.151.7.979

Bowlby, J. (1973). *Attachment and loss: Vol. 2. Separation.* New York, NY: Basic Books.

Brennan, K. A., Clark, C. L., & Shaver, P. R. (1998). Self-report measurement of adult romantic attachment: An integrative overview. In J. A. Simpson & W. S. Rhodes (Eds.), *Attachment theory and close relationships* (pp. 46–76). New York, NY: Guilford Press.

Browne, M. W., & Cudeck, R. (1992). Alternative ways of assessing model fit. *Sociological Methods & Research, 21*(2), 230–258. doi:10.1177/0049124192021002005

Bryant, P., & Dunford, R. (2008). The influence of regulatory focus on risky decision–making. *Applied Psychology, 57*(2), 335–359. doi:10.1111/j.1464-0597.2007.00319.x

Busemeyer, J. R., & Jones, L. E. (1983). Analysis of multiplicative combination rules when the causal variables are measured with error. *Psychological Bulletin, 93*(3), 549–562. doi:10.1037/0033-2909.93.3.549

Cameron, J. J., Finnegan, H., & Morry, M. M. (2012). Orthogonal dreams in an oblique world: A meta-analysis of the association between attachment anxiety and avoidance. *Journal of Research in Personality, 46*(5), 472–476. doi:10.1016/j.jrp.2012.05.001

Cann, A., Norman, M. A., Welbourne, J. L., & Calhoun, L. G. (2008). Attachment styles, conflict styles and humour styles: Interrelationships and associations with relationship satisfaction. *European Journal of Personality, 22,* 131–146. doi:10.1002/per.666

Cassidy, J. (2000). Adult romantic attachments: A development perspective on individual differences. *Review of General Psychology, 4*(2), 111–131. doi:10.1037/1089-2680.4.2.111

Cohen, J. (1992). Quantitative methods in psychology: A power primer. *Psychological Bulletin, 112*(1), 155–159. doi:10.1037/0033-2909.112.1.155

Chon, K. K., Choi, S-J., & Yang, B-C. (2001). Integrated adaptation of CES-D in Korea. *Korean Journal of Health Psychology, 6*(1), 59–76.

Chun, S., & Lee, K-H. (2008). The examination of path model among neuroticism, state anxiety, self-efficacy, and career exploration behavior: Based on the regulatory focus theory. *Korean Journal of Social and Personality Psychology, 22*(4), 93–110.

DeVito, C. C. (2014). *The link between insecure attachment and depression: Two potential pathways.* Unpublished master's thesis. Amherst, MA: The University of Massachusetts-Amherst.

Gnilka, P. B., Ashby, J. S., & Noble, C. M. (2013). Adaptive and maladaptive perfectionism as mediators of adult attachment styles and depression, hopelessness, and life satisfaction. *Journal of Counseling & Development, 91*(1), 78–86. doi:10.1002/j.1556-6676.2013.00074.x

Hair, J. F., Black, W. C., Babin, B. J., & Anderson, R. E. (2010). *Multivariate data analysis* (7th ed.). Upper Saddle River, NJ: Prentice Hall.

Hayes, A. F. (2013a). *Introduction to mediation, moderation, and conditional process analysis: A regression-based approach.* New York, NY: The Guilford Press.

Hayes, A. F. (2013b). The PROCESS macro for SPSS and SAS (version 2.13) [Software]. Retrieved from http://www.processmacro.org/download.html

Haws, K. L., Dholakia, U. M., & Bearden, W. O. (2010). An assessment of chronic regulatory focus measures. *Journal of Marketing Research, 47*(5), 967–982. doi:10.1509/jmkr.47.5.967

Health Insurance Review & Assessment Service. (2015). *Total medical care cost* [Healthcare Big Data Hub]. Retrieved from http://opendata.hira.or.kr/op/opc/olapJdgeChargeInfo.do.

Higgins, E. T. (1997). Beyond pleasure and pain. *American Psychologist, 52,* 1280–1300. doi:10.1037/0003-066X.52.12.1280

Higgins, E. T., & Roney, C. J. R., Crowe, E., & Hymes, C. (1994). Ideal versus ought predilections for approach and avoidance: Distinct self-regulatory systems. *Journal of Personality and Social Psychology, 66*(2), 276–286. doi:10.1037/0022-3514.66.2.276

Hu, L., & Bentler, P. M. (1999). Cutoff criteria for fit indexes in covariance structure analysis: Conventional criteria versus new alternatives. *Structural Equation Modeling, 6*(1), 1–55. doi:10.1080/10705519909540118

Jackman, M. G., Leite, W. L., & Cochrane, D. J. (2011). Estimating latent variable interactions with the unconstrained approach: A comparison of methods to form product indicators for large, unequal numbers of items. *Structural Equation Modeling, 18*(2), 274–288. doi:10.1080/10705511.2011.557342

Jinyao, Y., Xiongzhao, Z., Auerbach, R. P., Gardiner, C. K., Lin, C., Yuping, W., & Shuqiao, Y. (2012). Insecure attachment as a predictor of depressive and anxious symptomology. *Depression and Anxiety, 29*(9), 789–796. doi:10.1002/da.21953

Kim, S-H. (2004). *Adaptation of the experiences in close relationships-revised scale in to Korean: Confirmatory factor analysis and item response theory approaches.* Unpublished master's thesis. Seoul National University, Seoul, Korea.

Klenk, M. M., Strauman, T. J., & Higgins, E. T. (2011). Regulatory focus and anxiety: A self-regulatory model of GAD-depression comorbidity. *Personality and Individual Differences, 50*(7), 935–943. doi:10.1016/j.paid.2010.12.003

Lee, S., Baek, J., Yoon, Y., & Kim, J. (2013). A study on the socioeconomic impact and management of mental health problems: Focusing on Depression. (NHIS Report No. 2013–02). Seoul, ROK: National Health Insurance Service. Retrieved from Research on National Health Insurance Service website: http://www.nhis.or.kr/bbs7/boards/B0069/6682?boardKey=39&sort=sequence&order=desc&rows=10&messageCategoryKey=&pageNumber=1&viewType=generic&targetType=12&targetKey=39&status=&period=&startdt=&enddt=&queryField=T&query=2013-02

Little, T. D., Cunningham, W. A., Shahar, G., & Widaman, K. F. (2002). To parcel or not to parcel: Exploring the question, weighing the merits. *Structural Equation Modeling, 9*(2), 151–173. doi:10.1207/S15328007SEM0902_1

Lopez, F. G., & Brennan, K. A. (2000). Dynamic processes underlying adult attachment organization: Toward an attachment theoretical perspective on the healthy and effective self. *Journal of Counseling Psychology, 47*(3), 283–301. doi:10.1037/0022-0167.47.3.283

Marsh, H. W., Wen, Z. & Hau, K. T. (2004). Structural equation models of latent interactions: Evaluation of alternative estimation strategies and indicator construction. *Psychological Methods, 9*(3), 275–300. doi:10.1037/1082-989X.9.3.275

Mikulincer, M., & Shaver, P. R. (2003). The attachment behavioral system in adulthood: Activation, psychodynamics, and interpersonal processes. In M. Zanna (Ed.), *Advances in experimental social psychology* (Vol. *35*). New York, NY: Academic Press.

Myhr, G., Sookman, D., & Pinard, G. (2004). Attachment security and parental bonding in adults with obsessive-compulsive disorder: A comparison with depressed out-patients and healthy controls. *Acta Psychiatrica Scandinavica, 109*, 447–456. doi:10.1111/j.1600-0047.2004.00271.x

Ouschan, L., Boldero, J. M., Kashima, Y., Wakimoto, R., & Kashima, E. S. (2007). Regulatory focus strategies scale: A measure of individual differences in the endorsement of regulatory strategies. *Asian Journal of Social Psychology, 10*(4), 243–257. doi:10.1111/j.1467-839X.2007.00233.x

Park, J-E., & Lee, E-H. (2008). Adolescents' insecure attachments and problem behaviors: The moderating role of empathic ability. *The Korean Journal of Counseling and Psychotherapy, 20*(2), 369–389.

Pietromonaco, P. R., & Barrett, L. F. (1997). Working models of attachment and daily social interactions. *Journal of Personality and Social Psychology, 73*(6), 1409–1423. doi:10.1037/0022-3514.73.6.1409

Ponizovsky, A. M., & Drannikov, A. (2013). Contribution of attachment insecurity to health-related quality of life in depressed patients. *World Journal of Psychiatry, 3*(2), 41. doi:10.5498/wjp.v3.i2.41

Radloff, L. S. (1977). The CES-D Scale: A self-report depression scale for research in the general population. *Applied Psychological Measurement, 1*, 385–401. doi:10.1177/014662167700100306

Reis, S., & Grenyer, B. (2004). Fear of intimacy in women: Relationship between attachment styles and depressive symptoms. *Psychopathology, 37*, 299–303. doi:10.1159/000082268

Robert, J. E., Gotlib, I. H., & Kassel, J. D. (1996). Adult attachment security and symptoms of depression: The mediating roles of dysfunctional attitudes and low self-esteem. *Journal of Personality and Social Psychology*, *70*(2), 310–320. doi:10.1037/0022-3514.70.2.310

Safran, J. D. (1990). Towards a refinement of cognitive therapy in light of interpersonal theory: I. Theory. *Clinical Psychology Review*, *10*(1), 87–105. doi:10.1016/0272-7358(90)90108-M

Schokker, M. C., Links, T. P., Luttik, M. L., & Hagedoorn, M. (2010). The association between regulatory focus and distress in patients with a chronic disease: The moderating role of partner support. *British Journal of Health Psychology*, *15*(1), 63–78. doi:10.1348/135910709X429091

Semin, G. R., Higgins, T., de Montes, L. G., Estourget, Y., & Valencia, J. F. (2005). Linguistic signatures of regulatory focus: How abstraction fits promotion more than prevention. *Journal of Personality and Social Psychology*, *89*(1), 36–45. doi:10.1037/0022-3514.89.1.36

Simpson, J. A., & Rholes, W. S. (2004). Anxious attachment and depressive symptoms: An interpersonal perspective. In W. S. Rholes & J. A. Simpson (Eds.), *Adult attachment: Theory, research, and clinical implications* (pp. 408–437). New York, NY: Guilford Press

Ståhl, T., van Laar, C., & Ellemers, N. (2012). The role of prevention focus under stereotype threat: Initial cognitive mobilization is followed by depletion. *Journal of Personality and Social Psychology*, *102*(6), 1239. doi:10.1037/a0027678

Tabachinick, B. G., & Fidell, L. S. (2013). *Using multivariate statistics* (6th ed.). Boston, MA: Pearson.

Wallin, D. J. (2007). *Attachment in psychotherapy*. New York, NY: Guilford Press.

Wei, M., Heppner, P. P., Russell, D. W., & Young, S. K. (2006). Maladaptive perfectionism and ineffective coping as mediators between attachment and subsequent depression: A prospective analyses. *Journal of Counseling Psychology*, *53*, 67–79. doi:10.1037/0022-0167.53.1.67

Wei, M., Mallinckrodt, B., Larson, L. A., & Zakalik, R. A. (2005). Attachment, depression, and validation from self and others. *Journal of Counseling Psychology*, *52*, 368–377. doi:10.1037/0022-0167.52.3.368

Wei, M., Mallinckrodt, B., Russell, D. W., & Abraham, W. T. (2004). Maladaptive perfectionism as a mediator and moderator between adult attachment and depressive mood. *Journal of Counseling Psychology*, *51*(2), 201–212. doi:10.1037/0022-0167.51.2.201

Wei, M., Russell, D. W., & Zakalik, R. A. (2005). Adult attachment, social self-efficacy, self-disclosure, loneliness, and subsequent depression for freshman college students: A longitudinal study. *Journal of Counseling Psychology*, *52*(4), 602–614. doi:10.1037/0022-0167.52.4.602

Wei, M., Vogel, D. L., Ku, T., & Zakalik, R. A. (2005). Adult attachment, affect regulation, psychological distress, and interpersonal problems: The mediating role of emotional reactivity and emotional cutoff. *Journal of Counseling Psychology*, *52*, 14–24. doi:10.1037/0022-0167.52.1.14

Wen, Z., Marsh, H. W., & Hau, K. T. (2010). Structural equation models of latent interactions: An appropriate standardized solution and its scale-free properties. *Structural Equation Modeling*, *17* (1), 1–22. doi:10.1080/10705510903438872

Whisman, M. A., & McGarvey, A. L. (1995). Attachment, depressotypic cognitions, and dysphoria. *Cognitive Therapy and Research*, *19*(6), 633–650. doi:10.1007/BF02227858

The Role of Mindful Self-Care in the Relationship between Emotional Intelligence and Burnout in University Students

Natasha M. Loi and Nyree Pryce

ABSTRACT

Academic burnout can have serious consequences for university students. Students are prone to higher levels of stress and depression, poorer academic performance, and attrition from university. It is therefore important to investigate factors associated with these deleterious outcomes in order to assist educators develop effective programs to proactively address student well-being. The purpose of this study was to explore the associations between emotional intelligence (EI), student well-being, mindful self-care (MSC), and academic burnout. A further aim was to investigate the mediating role of MSC in the EI-burnout relationship. A sample of 216 university students (167 females; 78%) 18 years and older ($M = 35.57$, $SD = 11.59$) completed a battery of questionnaires associated with life satisfaction, EI, MSC, and academic burnout. Results found that EI was positively associated with well-being and MSC and negatively associated with each dimension of academic burnout. A series of multiple regression mediation analyses found that MSC mediated the relationship between EI and the exhaustion and efficacy dimensions of academic burnout. However, MSC did not mediate the relationship between EI and cynicism. The findings of this study suggest that MSC may be an important factor for improving student well-being and protecting against academic burnout.

The demand of engaging in tertiary education is inherently stressful and presents students with many challenges. When there are insufficient resources to cope with these demands, academic burnout may be the end result. Examining the factors related to academic burnout is an important area of research. Understanding both protective and potentiating factors may lead to the development of effective interventions to help reduce or prevent the incidence of academic burnout. Exploring the relationships of factors such as emotional intelligence, subjective well-being, and mindful self-care, provides insights into what may influence academic burnout, as well as the ways that students may handle the challenges of tertiary education.

The demands of coursework, the pressure to achieve, lack of sleep, adjustments to student life, and the associated financial, relationship, and life stress associated with tertiary study can result in negative outcomes including burnout (Houghton et al.,

2012; Lin & Huang, 2014). Research has found many university students experience high levels of psychological stress (Bayram & Bilgel, 2008; Fong & Loi, 2016). For example, in Australia, university students have been found to have greater levels of psychological distress than the general population (Stallman, 2010). For instance, Stallman (2010) found that 19% of the university students sampled scored in the very high stress range, compared to only 3% in the general population. Furthermore, Larcombe et al. (2016) found that students' responses on the Depression Anxiety Stress Scales (Lovibond & Lovibond, 1995) were substantially higher than general sample responses. Stress levels have also found to be high in postgraduate psychology students with 59 to 73% of students reporting clinically significant distress (Stafford-Brown & Pakenham, 2012). Prolonged or excessive stress can ultimately result in cynicism, disengagement, reduced efficacy, and increased emotional exhaustion, typical of academic burnout (Schaufeli et al., 2002).

The study of academic burnout warrants attention for many reasons. Burnout can have adverse effects on students' physical and mental well-being (Cazan & Năstasă, 2015; Lin & Huang, 2014). According to Lin and Huang (2014), academic burnout can result in a low sense of achievement, leading to negative attitudes, emotions, and behaviors toward learning. Furthermore, burnout can reduce motivation and result in poor academic outcomes (Beaumont et al., 2016). The consequences of academic burnout can be serious. Oswalt and Riddock (2007) found that academic burnout is strongly associated with higher levels of stress and depression, and an increased rate of suicidal ideation among students. An increased rate of attrition from university is also associated with academic burnout (Deary et al., 2003). Furthermore, burnout can have long-term consequences. For instance, Rudman and Gustavsson (2012) found that experiencing academic burnout was related to a reduced ability for students to master the occupational skills needed for tasks in the workforce in the first year proceeding graduation.

Because the prevalence, risk, and consequences of academic burnout are significant, investigation into more proactive approaches to address burnout in university students is needed, becoming more crucial in recent years. In 2008, in a review by the Australian government into higher education, recommendations were made to increase the proportion of 25 to 34-year-olds who hold a bachelor's degree by 2020 (Bradley et al., 2008). In 2020, the Australian government also announced that an extra 39,000 university places are to be created by 2023, and that 100,000 more places will be created by 2030, along with reductions in fees for some university courses (Tehan, 2020). These targeted approaches to increasing student numbers may also result in a greater number of students in Australian universities who will experience academic burnout. Therefore, research examining this particular population is of importance.

Academic Burnout

Academic burnout has been referred to as a psychological syndrome and has been defined by three key dimensions (Maslach & Leiter, 2016) including increased emotional exhaustion and cynicism and reduced efficacy (Maslach & Leiter, 2016). Emotional exhaustion has been described as fatigue, depletion, being worn out, and lacking in mental and physical energy (Cazan & Năstasă, 2015). Cynicism includes disengagement from studies, interpersonal distancing, a negative attitude, irritability, and a loss of idealism (Cazan & Năstasă, 2015; Maslach & Leiter, 2016). Efficacy, the belief that one has the capability to perform a certain task, is replaced with feelings of incompetence or a poor work standard in academic burnout (Cazan & Năstasă, 2015; Freire et al., 2020). Burnout may therefore occur due to a depletion of the resources needed to cope with stress (Cazan & Năstasă, 2015). Previous research has established that some of the correlates of academic burnout include emotional intelligence (Adeyemo, 2007), subjective well-being (Austin et al., 2005; Cazan & Năstasă, 2015), and mindful self-care (Cook-Cottone & Guyker, 2018; Feng et al., 2012).

Emotional Intelligence, Well-Being, and Mindful Self-Care

Emotional intelligence (EI) is defined by Salovey and Mayer (1990) as a set of emotional abilities that allows an individual to use information from their emotions to develop adaptive coping mechanisms. Their four-dimensional model includes perceiving emotions in oneself and others; understanding emotions in oneself and others; regulating emotions in oneself; and using emotions to guide thoughts and actions and to facilitate performance (Salovey et al., 2008). Alternatively, EI may be conceptualized as a combination of emotions related to self-perceptions, personality, and motivational traits and dispositions (Petrides et al., 2007). This type of noncognitive EI is best measured by self-report inventories (Zeidner et al., 2012). A model of EI including both ability and trait perspectives proposes that EI consists of emotional self-awareness as well as characteristics involving emotional regulation such as interpersonal, problem solving, and stress coping skills (Mayer et al., 2008). EI has been positively correlated with academic performance (Van der Zee et al., 2002), self-efficacy, workload, and social support (Yang, 2004), and psychological well-being (Ciarrochi et al., 2002), making EI an important variable of interest.

Ryan and Deci (2001) broadly define well-being in terms of subjective happiness, optimal individual functioning, and experience known as hedonic well-being. Diener (2000) defines well-being as the experience of positive affect and the absence of negative affect and an individual's sense of pleasure and satisfaction with life, also known as eudemonic well-being. The term *well-being* therefore, will refer to both psychological (eudemonic) and subjective (hedonic) components in the current study.

Self-care is operationalized as activities that promote physical and mental wellness and preserve health (Sünbül et al., 2018). For example, self-care practices may include eating a healthy diet, getting enough exercise, and engaging in activities that help to counteract stress, such as relaxation. In an extension of the self-care model, Cook-Cottone and Guyker (2018) included the element of *mindfulness* in a newly identified construct of mindful self-care (MSC). Mindfulness has been defined as awareness, in the present moment, of internal and external experiences (Brown & Ryan, 2003). When mindfulness is combined with self-care, it is defined by Cook-Cottone and Guyker (2018) as intentional engagement in self-care practices, with a mindful awareness of external demands and internal needs and how to meet those needs to improve physical and psychological well-being. The MSC model includes six subscales: (1) physical care (i.e.

engaging in healthy eating and exercising); (2) supportive relationships (i.e. choosing positive relations); (3) mindful awareness (i.e. an integrative and aligned attitude to internal and external experiences); (4) self-compassion and purpose (i.e. a kind and goal-orientated attitude toward the self); (5) mindful relaxation (i.e. activities to help relax with presence); and (6) supportive structure (i.e. a balance between environmental demands and forming a supportive strategy to meet them, for example, timetabling study; Cook-Cottone & Guyker, 2018).

Relationships between MSC and improved well-being have been established in student samples (e.g. Feng et al., 2019; Sünbül et al., 2018). As MSC integrates the intentional practice of self-care with mindful awareness of external and internal physiological and mental health needs (Cook-Cottone & Guyker, 2018), investigations using this holistic approach to self-care may have the potential to be particularly beneficial to students who are at high risk of stress.

As well as investigating the interrelationships of the factors associated with academic burnout (i.e. student well-being and EI), and given that MSC has been found to be associated with student well-being (Feng et al., 2019), and the practice of MSC is considered protective against the onset of mental health symptoms and burnout (Hotchkiss & Lesher, 2018), a further aim of the current study was to examine the novel extension of the self-care research and examine whether MSC mediates the relationship between EI and academic burnout.

Interrelationships between Academic Burnout, Well-Being, EI and MSC

Applying existing models such as the jobs demands-resources theory (Demerouti et al., 2001) and the conservation of resources theory (Hobfoll, 1989) in an academic context, burnout can be viewed as the result of an imbalance between the demands of university study and a lack of resources to adequately cope with these demands (Alarcon et al., 2011; Leupold et al., 2020). Austin et al. (2005) suggested that EI can enhance resources to cope with demands and that individuals who are high in EI are more skilled at expressing, understanding, and regulating emotions. Thus, they are able to cope with the stress and hassles of everyday life. The fact that individuals with high EI appraise environmental stressors as challenges is proposed to be the mechanism by which psychological stress is managed (Zeidner et al., 2012). The EI dimension of self-emotion appraisal was found to be related to decreased burnout in a study by Carvalho et al. (2018), suggesting that individuals who are adept at understanding and communicating their emotions are less prone to the negative effects of chronic stress. Previous findings by Cazan and Năstasă (2015) have also established the positive relationship between EI and life satisfaction and the negative relationship between EI and burnout, as well as the mediating role of burnout in the EI-life satisfaction relationship.

Previous research has proposed a relationship between well-being, mindfulness, and EI. Mindfulness has been linked to the development of emotional regulation; one of the dimensions of EI (Koole, 2009). Schutte and Malouff (2011) investigated the relationship between the three constructs and suggested that the core attentional and non-judgmental aspects of mindfulness may encourage individuals to develop better emotional regulation and general EI, leading to increased well-being. A study by

Enríquez et al. (2017) adds further support to the mindfulness-EI relationship. In an experiment using a mindfulness intervention, pre- and post-test scores two months apart were obtained from self-report questionnaires measuring burnout, engagement, emotional regulation, empathy, and personality traits. The results of this study found that mindfulness training can increase EI, decrease anxiety and burnout, and improve emotional regulation (Enríquez et al., 2017). This result suggests that the combination of mindfulness and EI can positively impact well-being and enhance the resources needed to cope with demands.

Another of the processes by which EI may be associated with well-being is as a facilitator of positive health practices including self-care such as through regular exercise and a healthy diet (Zeidner et al., 2012). Components of self-care include self-compassion (Neely et al., 2009) and self-kindness (Stallman et al., 2018). In an academic context, these components of self-care may be lacking when students are hard on themselves for falling below their own expectations, a practice that is detrimental to well-being (Neely et al., 2009). Self-care practices that may be facilitated by higher EI and mindfulness may enhance self-kindness and self-compassion leading to increased student well-being.

Self-care and mindfulness are also key components in the MSC model. Dimensions of MSC, such as seeking social support, eating healthily, and exercising regularly, have also been linked to EI (Zeidner et al., 2012). Preliminary research findings suggest MSC is positively associated with psychological well-being, especially the dimensions of mindful relaxation and self-compassion (Feng et al., 2019). Support for MSC as a preventative for burnout is offered by Sünbül et al. (2018). The results of their study examining 262 undergraduate students found that all of the MSC dimensions significantly predicted well-being with supportive structure providing the greatest contribution. Research by Zahniser et al. (2017) found that the self-care practices of students helped to mitigate the detrimental effects of stress and resulted in improved well-being. Students in this study particularly benefited from self-care measures that improved support systems and awareness of their needs and reactions to stress. These aspects are aligned with the dimensions of the MSC model and add support to the importance of self-care.

The Current Study

Previous research maintains that both EI and MSC are factors associated with improved well-being. Therefore, drawing on previous findings, it is plausible that high levels of EI will result in better self-care practices and that these practices may benefit student well-being (Feng et al., 2019; Sünbül et al., 2018; Zahniser et al., 2017; Zeidner et al., 2012).

There is little research to date on the impact of MSC and the incidence of academic burnout. The current study, therefore, aimed to examine the relationships between dimensions of academic burnout (exhaustion, cynicism, and efficacy) and EI and MSC in a sample of Australian university students. Given the current empirical support for the relationships between these constructs, the current study aimed to investigate whether EI and MSC are related to academic burnout with the following specific hypotheses:

Hypothesis 1. EI would be positively associated with student well-being.

Hypothesis 2. EI would be positively associated with MSC.

Hypothesis 3. EI would be negatively associated with all dimensions of academic burnout.

Hypothesis 4. MSC would mediate the EI-burnout relationship, specifically each dimension of academic burnout, (exhaustion, cynicism, and efficacy).

Method

Participants

A power analysis was conducted using G*Power 3.1 (Faul et al., 2009). Assuming a medium effect size of $f^2 = .15$, a critical alpha level of .05, and a power level of .90, the power analysis indicated that a minimum of 123 participants were required.

Participants consisted of English-speaking students, aged 18 years and older recruited from a regional university in New South Wales, Australia. A total of 264 students accessed the survey, however, 49 were excluded as a result of significant missing data, yielding a final sample of 216 participants. The sample consisted of 47 males (22.0%) and 167 females (78.0%). Two students declined to specify gender. Participants ranged in age from 18 to 72 years ($M = 35.57$, $SD = 11.59$). The majority of participants were in their first year ($n = 115$; 53.5%), studying either Psychology ($n = 87$; 40.5%) or Law ($n = 70$; 32.6%).

Measures

Demographics

Participants were asked to provide information on their age, gender, course currently being studied, years of study, and marital and employment status.

Emotional Intelligence

The Assessing Emotions Scale (AES; Schutte et al., 1998) was used to assess EI. The scale is a 33-item self-report inventory measured on a 5-point Likert scale ranging from 1 (*strongly disagree*) to 5 (*strongly agree*). An example item is "I am aware of my emotions as I experience them". High scores indicate a higher degree of EI. The internal reliability for the current study was $\alpha = .93$.

Academic Burnout

The Maslach Burnout Inventory - General Survey for Students (MBI-SS; Schaufeli et al., 2002) is a 15-item measure, used to assess academic burnout in students on a 6-point scale ranging from 0 (*never*) to 5 (*very often*). Three subscales measure the following dimensions: exhaustion (5 items, e.g. "I feel emotionally drained by my studies"); cynicism (4 items, e.g. "I have become more cynical about the potential usefulness of my studies"), and efficacy (6 items), e.g. "During class I feel confident that I am effective in getting things done"). High scores on exhaustion and cynicism and low scores on efficacy are indicative of academic burnout. Internal reliability for the current study was good (exhaustion $\alpha = .93$; cynicism $\alpha = .90$; and efficacy $\alpha = .80$).

Mindful Self-Care

The Mindful Self-Care Scale (MSCS; Cook-Cottone & Guyker, 2018) is a 33-item self-report scale used to measure frequency of self-care behaviors on a 5-point Likert scale ranging from 1 (*never – 0 days*) to 5 (*regularly – 6-7 days*). Questions are answered based on the frequency of occurrence in the last week. The measure includes six subscales: physical care (e.g. "I exercised at least 30 to 60 min"); supportive relationships (e.g. "I felt supported by people in my life"); mindful awareness (e.g. "I had a calm awareness of my feelings"); self-compassion and purpose (e.g. "I kindly acknowledged my own challenges and difficulties"); mindful relaxation (e.g. "I did something creative to relax"), and supportive structure (e.g. "I maintained balance between the demands of others and what is important to me"). High scores are indicative of better self-care. The internal reliability for this study was α = .90.

Well-Being

Subjective well-being was measured using the Satisfaction With Life Scale (SWLS; Diener et al., 1985). This 5-item scale measures global life satisfaction on a 7-point Likert scale ranging from 1 (*strongly disagree*) to 7 (*strongly agree*). An example of an item on this scale is, "I am satisfied with my life". High scores indicate greater life satisfaction. Internal reliability for the current sample was α = .87.

Procedure

The study was conducted after approval was granted from the host university's Human Research Ethics Committee (HE20-048). The online survey battery was delivered *via* Qualtrics™ software (Provo, UT). Participants were recruited by contacting Heads of Schools of a number of faculties within the host university to request that they share a link to a survey with their students. First year Psychology students were also recruited and received course credit for their participation. Participants were also recruited *via* word of mouth, and messages posted on university social media sites (e.g. Facebook). Upon accessing the survey, participants were asked to read an information sheet detailing the purpose of the study, potential risks, and the confidentiality of their responses. Participants were also informed that they could withdraw from the survey at any time. They were then asked to provide implied consent and proceed to the questionnaires. Participants were presented with the demographic questions first, followed by the questionnaires presented in the subsequent order: SWSL, MSCS, AES, and MBI-SS. The survey took approximately 25 min to complete.

Results

Statistical Analysis

All statistical analyses were conducted using SPSS v. 27. Pearson correlation coefficients were calculated to assess hypotheses 1 to 3. Hypothesis 4 was assessed using model 4 of the PROCESS macro for SPSS (Hayes, 2018).

Table 1. Descriptive Statistics and Bivariate Correlations for Main Study Variables (N = 216).

	1	2	3	4	5	6	7
1.Age	–						
2.Wellbeing	.07	–					
3.MSC	.12	.39***	–				
4.EI	.26***	.36***	.56***	–			
5.Exhaustion	−.28***	-.20**	-.31***	-.31***	–		
6.Cynicism	-.19**	-.17*	-.21**	-.23**	.73***	–	
7.Efficacy	-.20**	-.29***	-.52***	-.47***	.39***	.38***	–
M	35.57	23.16	18.30	124.94	11.52	5.71	9.37
SD	11.59	6.60	3.77	18.37	6.22	5.27	4.90
Range	18-72	5-35	9.53-27.34	45-159	0-25	0-20	0-23

$*p < .05$, $**p < .01$, $***p < .001$.

Descriptive Statistics and Bivariate Correlation Analyses

Means, standard deviations, and correlations for key variables are presented in Table 1. As predicted, a positive correlation was found between EI and student well-being, supporting hypothesis 1. A large positive relationship was found between EI and MSC thus supporting hypothesis 2. Hypothesis 3 was also supported with negative correlations found between EI and all three dimensions of burnout. This result indicates that EI was found to be significantly associated with increased levels of exhaustion and cynicism, and reduced efficacy.

Mediation Analyses

A series of multiple regression mediation analyses were conducted to test the hypothesis that MSC would mediate the relationship between EI and each dimension of academic burnout. Indirect effects for all mediation analysis were estimated using 95% bias-corrected bootstrapping based on 5000 replications.

In all mediation models, EI was a significant predictor of MSC. As shown in Figure 1, EI and MSC both significantly predicted exhaustion. The results of this analysis supports the hypothesis that MSC mediates the relationship between EI and exhaustion.

As shown in Figure 2, neither EI nor MSC were significant predictors of cynicism. Therefore, this analysis did not support the hypothesis that MSC would mediate the relationship between EI and cynicism.

Finally, as shown in Figure 3, both EI and MSC were significant predictors of reduced efficacy. The results of this analysis provides support for the hypothesis that MSC mediates the relationship between EI and reduced efficacy.

Discussion

The objective of this study was to investigate the interrelationships between EI, student well-being, MSC, and the academic burnout dimensions of exhaustion, cynicism, and reduced efficacy. Providing insight into the factors that may help to reduce stress, increase well-being, and prevent academic burnout has implications for students, educators, and institutions. As such, sustained research focus in required in order to mitigate the negative affects associated with university study. The relatively recent

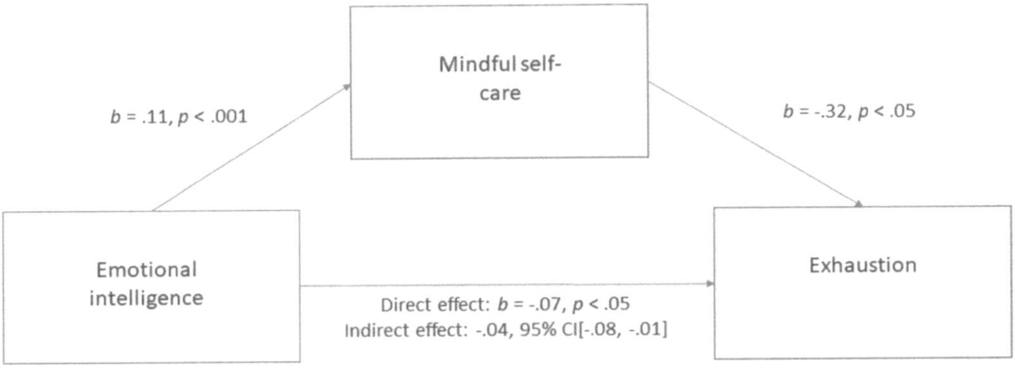

Figure 1. The mediating role of mindful self-care between emotional intelligence and exhaustion. *Note.* b = unstandardized regression coefficients; CI = bootstrapped confidence intervals based on 5000 samples.

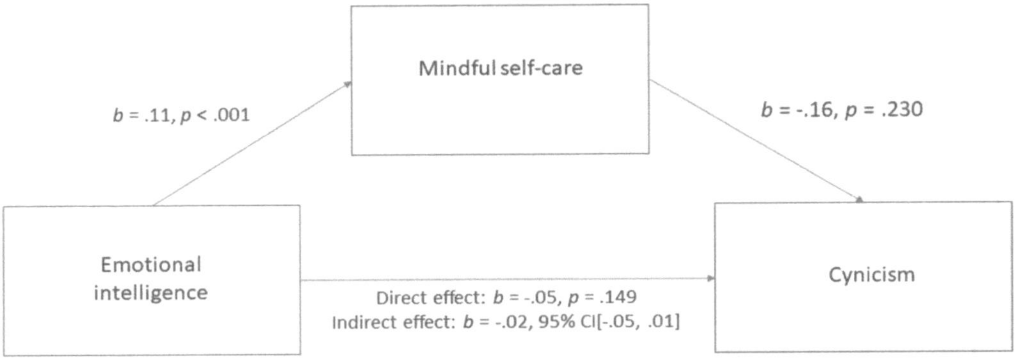

Figure 2. The mediation model showing no significant direct or indirect effects of mindful self-care on the relationship between emotional intelligence and cynicism. *Note.* b = unstandardized regression coefficients; CI = bootstrapped confidence intervals based on 5000 samples.

concept of MSC (Cook-Cottone & Guyker, 2018) provides a novel mechanism by which university students may be assisted to progress more confidently and positively through their education journey. As little research has examined the relationship between MSC and academic burnout, the current study aimed to provide some insight into the potential utility of MSC and the factors related to academic burnout in this population.

In accordance with the first three hypotheses, EI correlated positively with student well-being and MSC, and negatively with all dimensions of academic burnout. These findings are consistent with previous research suggesting that high EI is associated with low levels of student stress and burnout and enhanced psychological well-being (Cazan & Năstasă, 2015). These associations may potentially be explained by those with high EI using awareness, emotional expression, and emotional regulation adopt healthier responses to stress and view stressors as challenges rather than problems (Zeidner et al., 2012). Additionally, high EI has been linked to improvements in an

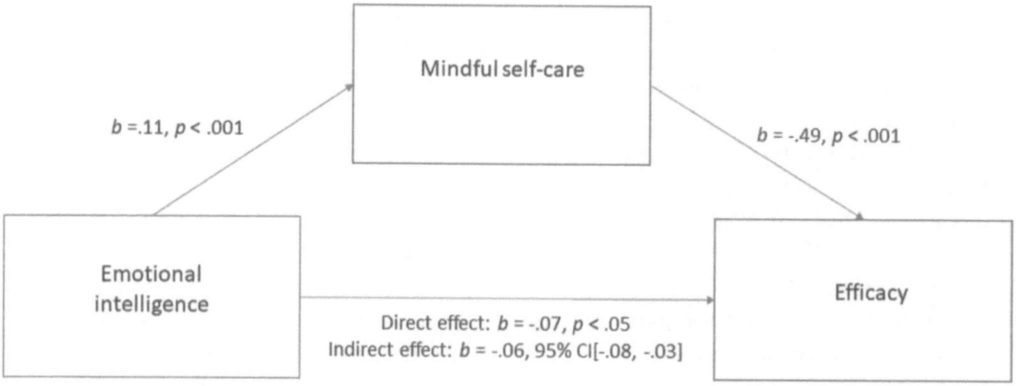

Figure 3. The mediating role of mindful self-care between emotional intelligence and efficacy. *Note.* b = unstandardized regression coefficients; CI = bootstrapped confidence intervals based on 5000 samples.

individual's ability to cope with demands and pressures (Cazan & Năstasă, 2015), which also accounts for reduced stress-related burnout.

The current study found a large positive association between EI and MSC. This is consistent with previous research that has found that high EI is associated with engagement in self-care practices (e.g. Testa & Sanggamjanavanich, 2016) and mindfulness (Schutte & Malouff, 2011). These findings suggest that high EI is linked to a greater tendency to practice self-care with mindful intention, such as eating a healthy diet, exercising, engaging in activities for relaxation, and seeking supportive relationships. Furthermore, research has theorized that mindfulness can improve EI (Enríquez et al., 2017) and that self-care training can also increase EI in students (Goudarzian et al., 2019). These previous findings, in combination with results from the current study, imply that the interrelationships between EI, well-being, and MSC have the potential to result in a greater tendency to practice MSC, and that the practice of MSC may result in enhanced EI. Both of these factors are associated with improved student well-being and the reduction of academic burnout (Goudarzian et al., 2019; Sünbül et al., 2018). Previous research has also found that EI as well as self-care skills can be learned (Goudarzian et al., 2019; Testa & Sanggamjanavanich, 2016). Students who are taught EI and MSC early in their academic careers may then be better equipped to cope with the challenges of tertiary education, have improved academic outcomes, maintain their physical and psychological health, and experience greater success in their careers through the prevention of academic burnout.

The hypothesis that MSC would mediate the relationship between EI and the three components of academic burnout was partially supported. MSC was found to mediate the relationship between EI and exhaustion and reduced efficacy. These findings are somewhat consistent with previous research that has found MSC is linked to decreased burnout (Hotchkiss & Lesher, 2018; Sünbül et al., 2018). Of all the dimensions of academic burnout, MSC provided the greatest protection against reduced efficacy. This finding suggests that MSC has an important role in preserving students' beliefs about their ability to competently fulfill academic challenges. Efficacy is an important determinant of student well-being, success, and academic achievement (Freire et al., 2020). Therefore, strategies that utilize MSC during university study can help to protect students' self-efficacious beliefs, and lead to a proficient and psychologically healthy student body.

MSC also accounted for significant protection against exhaustion. This suggests that MSC plays an important role in helping to maintain students' physical health. MSC strategies that help to prevent exhaustion can help prevent students feeling drained by their studies and help to sustain their physical health, thus leading to improved academic outcomes.

However, MSC did not mediate the relationship between EI and cynicism, suggesting that the practice of self-care may be more relevant to alleviating physical symptoms of burnout (i.e. exhaustion – feeling emotionally drained, tired, burned out) as well as acting as a protective factor against reduced efficacy (e.g. feeling incapable of undertaking and succeeding in tasks). The sense of detachment or indifference evident in the cynicism dimension is antithetical to the components of MSC which assess, for instance, mindful awareness, self-compassion and purpose, and mindful relaxation (Cook-Cottone & Guyker, 2018).

Overall, the results of the current study provide evidence of the interrelationships between EI, student well-being, MSC, and academic burnout and that MSC may be a major factor in the relationship between EI and two dimensions of burnout. These findings are consistent with previous research suggesting that EI and self-care can assist in improving psychological well-being and that extending the self-care model to include mindfulness may have a protective effect against academic burnout in university students (Cazan & Năstasă, 2015; Schutte & Malouff, 2011; Sünbül et al., 2018). Using the jobs demands-resources theory (Demerouti et al., 2001) and the conservation of resources theory (Hobfoll, 1989), MSC can be viewed as an investment in building resources to help cope with stress to help prevent academic burnout. Furthermore, the steady and intentional practice of MSC, suggested by Cook-Cottone and Guyker (2018) may be a factor that is protective against academic burnout.

According to Cook-Cottone and Guyker (2018), self-care is foundational for physical and emotional well-being. Students are prone to experiencing high levels of stress that can negatively impact their physical and emotional well-being and potentially lead to academic burnout (e.g. Bayram & Bilgel, 2008; Fong & Loi, 2016; Lin & Huang, 2014). Therefore, these findings have important implications for academic institutions who can proactively implement strategies utilizing MSC to improve student well-being. The development of preventative MSC education and interventions integrated into the curriculum may serve to reduce or prevent academic burnout by preserving self-efficacious beliefs and preventing exhaustion.

Limitations and Future Research

Some limitations of the current study should be noted. Conclusions about causality among key variables are limited by the correlational design of the current study. The use of self-report measures in the current study are open to bias. The convenience sample of predominantly female students from one Australian rural university campus limits the generalizability of findings. Additionally, the current sample consisted

predominantly of Psychology students who may have inherently higher levels of EI due to their helping nature as suggested by Testa and Sanggamjanavanich (2016). Finally, participants in the current sample had a high level of well-being at the outset of the study.

The influence of other contributing variables such as motivational style and personality traits has not been ruled out. These variables have also been closely linked to concepts in the current study such as efficacy and burnout (Ariani, 2017). Including variables such as these could help provide greater insight into the mechanisms underlying academic burnout and would be an interesting area for future research. Other areas for future research may include investigation of each dimension of MSC as individual variables to examine the elements of the MSC model that have the greatest impact on academic burnout. Research using experimental designs to assess the effectiveness of MSC interventions is also an important area for future study.

Conclusion

University study presents students with a unique set of stressors. This leaves students vulnerable to high levels of psychological stress that can negatively impact their physical and psychological well-being. As a result of high stress levels, students are at increased risk of mental health disorders and academic burnout. Evidence of the interrelationships between EI, student well-being, MSC, and academic burnout were confirmed in the current study. It is among the first to establish these relationships in an Australian university student sample using the novel construct of MSC, and to examine the mediating role of MSC in the EI academic burnout relationship. Since university students are at high risk of academic burnout, it is important to identify factors that may reduce or prevent its occurrence. Creating targeted MSC interventions that promote and develop intentional engagement in self-care may result in improvements in student well-being, thus reducing or preventing the incidence of academic burnout. Ultimately, reducing academic burnout should be a priority for academic institutions given the positive outcomes which would likely result from a less stressed student body, including increased engagement with study and enhanced academic performance (e.g. improved grades). As such, the development of practices that utilize MSC presents an actionable opportunity for universities.

Funding

The author(s) reported there is no funding associated with the work featured in this article.

References

Adeyemo, D. A. (2007). Moderating influence of emotional intelligence on the link between academic self-efficacy and achievement of university students. *Psychology and Developing Societies*, *19*(2), 199–213. https://doi.org/0.1177/097133360701900204

Alarcon, G. M., Edwards, J. M., & Menke, L. E. (2011). Student burnout and engagement: A test of the conservation of resources theory. *The Journal of Psychology*, *145*(3), 211–227. https://doi.org/10.1080/00223980.2011.555432

Ariani, D. W. (2017). Why am I burnout and engaged? The role of motivation and personality. *Journal of Psychological and Educational Research*, *25*, 61–89. https://www.proquest.com/docview/1964017748?pq-origsite=gscholar&fromopenview=true

Austin, E. J., Saklofske, D. H., & Egan, V. (2005). Personality, well-being, and health correlates of trait emotional intelligence. *Personality and Individual Differences*, *38*(3), 547–558. https://doi.org/10.1016/j.paid.2004.05.009

Bayram, N., & Bilgel, N. (2008). The prevalence and socio-demographic correlations of depression, anxiety and stress among a group of university students. *Social Psychiatry and Psychiatric Epidemiology*, *43*(8), 667–672. https://doi.org/10.1007/s00127-008-0345-x

Beaumont, E., Durkin, M., Hollins Martin, C. J., & Carson, J. (2016). Compassion for others, self-compassion, quality of life and mental well-being measures and their association with compassion fatigue and burnout in student midwives: A quantitative survey. *Midwifery*, *34*, 239–244. https://doi.org/10.1016/j.midw.2015.11.002

Bradley, D. B., Noonan, P., Nugent, H., & Scales, B. (2008). *Australian government review of higher education: Final report [Bradley review]*. Department of Education, Employment, and Workplace Relations. http://hdl.voced.edu.au/10707/44384

Brown, K. W., & Ryan, R. M. (2003). The benefits of being present: Mindfulness and its role in psychological well-being. *Journal of Personality and Social Psychology*, *84*(4), 822–848. https://doi.org/10.1037/0022-3514.84.4.822

Carvalho, V. S., Guerrero, E., & Chambel, M. J. (2018). Emotional intelligence and health students' well-being: A two-wave study with students of medicine, physiotherapy and nursing. *Nurse Education Today*, *63*, 35–42. https://doi.org/0.1016/j.nedt.2018.01.010

Cazan, A.-M., & Năstasă, L. E. (2015). Emotional intelligence, satisfaction with life and burnout among university students. *Procedia - Social and Behavioral Sciences*, *180*, 1574–1578. https://doi.org/10.1016j.sbspro.2015.02.309

Ciarrochi, J., Deane, F. P., & Anderson, S. (2002). Emotional intelligence moderates the relationship between stress and mental health. *Personality and Individual Differences*, *32*(2), 197–209. https://doi.org/10.1016/S0191-8869(01)00012-5

Cook-Cottone, C. P., & Guyker, W. M. (2018). The development and validation of the Mindful Self-Care Scale (MSCS): An assessment of practices that support positive embodiment. *Mindfulness*, *9*(1), 161–175. https://doi.org/10.1007/s12671-017-0759-1

Deary, I. J., Watson, R., & Hogston, R. (2003). A longitudinal cohort study of burnout and attrition in nursing students. *Journal of Advanced Nursing*, *43*(1), 71–81. https://doi.org/10.1046/j.1365-2648.2003.02674.x

Demerouti, E., Bakker, A. B., Nachreiner, F., & Schaufeli, W. B. (2001). The job-demands-resources model of burnout. *Journal of Applied Psychology*, *86*(3), 499–512. https://doi.org/10.1037//0021-9010.86.3.499

Diener, E. (2000). Subjective well-being: The science of happiness and a proposal for a national index. *American Psychologist*, *55*(1), 34–43. https://doi.org/10.1037/0003-066X.55.1.34

Diener, E., Emmons, R. A., Larsen, R. J., & Griffin, S. (1985). The satisfaction with life scale. *Journal of Personality Assessment*, *49*(1), 71–75. https://doi.org/10.1207/s15327752jpa4901_13

Enríquez, H., Ramos, N., & Esparza, O. (2017). Impact of the mindful emotional intelligence program on emotional regulation in college students. *International Journal of Psychology and Psychological Therapy*, *17*, 39–48. https://www.redalyc.org/pdf/560/56049624002.pdf

Faul, F., Erdfelder, E., Buchner, A., & Lang, A.-G. (2009). Statistical power analyses using G*Power 3.1: Tests for correlation and regression analyses. *Behavior Research Methods*, *41*(4), 1149–1160. https://doi.org/10.3758/BRM.41.4.11

Feng, X., Mosimah, C. I., Sizemore, G., Goyat, R., & Dwibedi, N. (2019). Impact of mindful self-care and perceived stress on the health-related quality of life among young-adult students in West Virginia. *Journal of Human Behavior in the Social Environment*, *29*(1), 26–36. https://doi.org/10.1080/10911359.2018.1470953

Feng, K., Zhao, J., & You, X. (2012). Emotional intelligence and life satisfaction in Chinese university students: The mediating role of self-esteem and social support. *Personality and Individual Differences*, *53*(8), 1039–1043. https://doi.org/10.1016/j.paid.2012.07.032

Fong, M., & Loi, N. M. (2016). The mediating role of self-compassion in student psychological health. *Australian Psychologist*, *51*(6), 431–441. https://doi.org/10.1111/ap.12185

Freire, C., Ferradás, M. D. M., Regueiro, B., Rodríguez, S., Valle, A., & Núñez, J. C. (2020). Coping strategies and self-efficacy in university students: A Person-Centered Approach. *Frontiers in Psychology*, *11*, 841. https://doi.org/10.3389/fpsyg.2020.00841

Goudarzian, A. H., Nesami, M. B., Sedghi, P., Gholami, M., Faraji, M., & Hatkehlouei, M. B. (2019). The effect of self-care education on emotional intelligence of Iranian nursing students: A quasi-experimental study. *Journal of Religion and Health*, *58*(2), 589–598. https://doi.org/10.1007/s10943-017-0537-3

Hayes, A. F. (2018). *Introduction to mediation, moderation and conditional process analysis: A regression-based approach* (2nd ed.). Guilford Press.

Hobfoll, S. E. (1989). Conservation of resources: A new attempt at conceptualizing stress. *American Psychologist*, *44*(3), 513–524. https://doi.org/10.1037//0003-066X.44.3.513

Hotchkiss, J. T., & Lesher, R. (2018). Factors predicting burnout among chaplains: Compassion satisfaction, organizational factors, and the mediators of mindful self-care and secondary traumatic stress. *Journal of Pastoral Care & Counseling*, *72*(2), 86–98. https://doi.org/10.1177/1542305018780655

Houghton, J. D., Wu, J., Godwin, J. L., Neck, C. P., & Manz, C. C. (2012). Effective stress management: A model of emotional intelligence, self-leadership, and student stress coping. *Journal of Management Education*, *36*(2), 220–238. https://doi.org/10.1177/1052562911430205

Koole, S. L. (2009). The psychology of emotion regulation: An integrative review. *Cognition & Emotion*, *23*(1), 4–41. https://doi.org/10.1080/02699930802619031

Larcombe, W., Finch, S., Sore, R., Murray, C. M., Kentish, S., Mulder, R. A., Lee-Stecum, P., Baik, C., Tokatlidis, O., & Williams, D. A. (2016). Prevalence and socio-demographic correlates of psychological distress among students at an Australian university. *Studies in Higher Education*, *41*(6), 1074–1091. https://doi.org/10.1080/03075079.2014.966072

Leupold, C. R., Lopina, E. C., & Erickson, J. (2020). Examining the effects of core self-evaluations and perceived organizational support on academic burnout among undergraduate students. *Psychological Reports*, *123*(4), 1260–1281. https://doi.org/10.1177/0033294119852767

Lin, S.-H., & Huang, Y.-C. (2014). Life stress and academic burnout. *Active Learning in Higher Education*, *15*(1), 77–90. https://doi.org/10.1177/1469787413514651

Lovibond, S. H., & Lovibond, P. F. (1995). *Manual for the depression anxiety stress scales*. 2nd ed., Psychology Foundation of Australia.

Maslach, C., & Leiter, M. P. (2016). Understanding the burnout experience: Recent research and its implications for psychiatry. *World Psychiatry : Official Journal of the World Psychiatric Association (WPA)*, *15*(2), 103–111. https://doi.org/10.1002/wps.20311

Mayer, J. D., Roberts, R. D., & Barsade, S. G. (2008). Human abilities: Emotional intelligence. *Annual Review of Psychology*, *59*, 507–536. https://doi.org/10.1146/annurev.psych.59.103006.093646

Neely, M. E., Schallert, D. L., Mohammed, S. S., Roberts, R. M., & Chen, Y. (2009). Self-kindness when facing stress: The role of self-compassion, goal regulation, and support in college students' well-being. *Motivation and Emotion*, *33*(1), 88–97. https://doi.org/10.1007/s11031-008-9119-8

Oswalt, S. B., Riddock, C. C. (2007). What to do about being overwhelmed: Graduate students, stress and university services. *College Student Affairs Journal*, *27*, 24–44. https://files.eric.ed.gov/fulltext/EJ899402.pdf

Petrides, K. V., Pérez-González, J. C., & Furnham, A. (2007). On the criterion and incremental validity of trait emotional intelligence. *Cognition & Emotion*, *21*(1), 26–55. https://doi.org/10.1080/02699930601038912

Rudman, A., & Gustavsson, J. P. (2012). Burnout during nursing education predicts lower occupational preparedness and future clinical performance: A longitudinal study. *International Journal of Nursing Studies*, *49*(8), 988–1001. https://doi.org/0.1016/j.ijnurstu.2012.03.010

Ryan, R. M., & Deci, E. L. (2001). On happiness and human potentials: A review of research on hedonic and eudaimonic well-being. *Annual Review of Psychology*, *52*, 141–166. https://doi.org/10.1146/annurev.psych.52.1.141

Salovey, P., & Mayer, J. D. (1990). Emotional intelligence. *Imagination, Cognition and Personality*, *9*(3), 185–211. https://doi.org/10.2190/DUGG-P24E-52WK-6CDG

Salovey, P., Mayer, J. D., & Caruso, D. R. (2008). Emotional intelligence: New ability or eclectic traits? *The American Psychologist*, *63*(6), 503–517. https://doi.org/10.1037/0003-066X.63.6.503

Schaufeli, W. B., Martinez, I. M., Marques Pinto, A., Salanova, M., & Bakker, A. B. (2002). Burnout and engagement in university students: A cross-national study. *Journal of Cross-Cultural Psychology*, *33*(5), 464–481. https://doi.org/10.1177/0022022102033005003

Schutte, N. S., & Malouff, J. M. (2011). Emotional intelligence mediates the relationship between mindfulness and subjective well-being. *Personality and Individual Differences*, *50*(7), 1116–1119. https://doi.org/10.1016/j.paid.2011.01.037

Schutte, N. S., Malouff, J. M., Hall, L. E., Haggerty, D. J., Cooper, J. T., Golden, C. J., & Dornheim, L. (1998). Development and validation of a measure of emotional intelligence. *Personality and Individual Differences*, *25*(2), 167–177. https://doi.org/10.1016/S0191-8869(98)00001-4

Stafford-Brown, J., & Pakenham, K. I. (2012). The effectiveness of an ACT informed intervention for managing stress and improving therapist qualities in clinical psychology trainees. *Journal of Clinical Psychology*, *68*(6), 592–613. https://doi.org/10.1002/jclp.21844

Stallman, H. M. (2010). Psychological distress in university students: A comparison with general population data. *Australian Psychologist*, *45*(4), 249–257. https://doi.org/10.1080/00050067.2010.482109

Stallman, H. M., Ohan, J. L., & Chiera, B. (2018). The role of social support, being present and self-kindness in university student well-being. *British Journal of Guidance & Counselling*, *46*(4), 365–374. https://doi.org/10.1080/03069885.2017.1343458

Sünbül, Z. A., Malkoç, A., Gördesli, M. A., Arslan, R., & Çekici, F. (2018). Mindful self-care dimensions as agents of well-being for students in mental health fields. *European Journal of Education Studies*, *5*, 33–41. https://doi.org/10.5281/zenodo.1469675

Tehan, D. (2020, June 19). *Minister for Education Dan Tehan National Press Club address*. https://ministers.dese.gov.au/tehan/minister-education-dan-tehan-national-press-club-address

Testa, D., & Sangganjanavanich, V. F. (2016). Contribution of mindfulness and emotional intelligence to burnout among counseling interns. *Counselor Education and Supervision*, *55*(2), 95–108. https://doi.org/10.1002/ceas.12035

Van der Zee, K., Thijs, M., & Schakel, L. (2002). The relationship of emotional intelligence with academic intelligence and the big five. *European Journal of Personality*, *16*(2), 103–125. https://doi.org/10.1002/per.434

Yang, H. (2004). Factors affecting student burnout and academic achievement in multiple enrolment programs in Taiwan's technical-vocational colleges. *International Journal of Educational Development*, *24*(3), 283–301. https://doi.org/10.1016/j.ijedudev.2003.12.001

Zahniser, E., Rupert, P. A., & Dorociak, K. E. (2017). Self-care in clinical psychology graduate training. *Training and Education in Professional Psychology*, *11*(4), 283–289. https://doi.org/10.1037/tep0000172

Zeidner, M., Matthews, G., & Roberts, R. D. (2012). The emotional intelligence, health, and well-being nexus: What have we learned and what have we missed? *Applied Psychology. Health and Well-Being*, *4*(1), 1–30. https://doi.org/10.1111/j.1758-0854.2011.01062.x

The Psychology of Health and Illness: The Mental Health and Physiological Effects of Intimate Partner Violence on Women

Nancy Lutwak

ABSTRACT
Violence against women is a global public health problem with about one in three women experiencing either physical and or sexual intimate partner violence during their lifetime. Globally as many as 38% of homicides committed against women are by a male intimate partner. Violence against women may have negative effects on their mental, physical, and reproductive health (WHO fact sheet, 2016). Untreated individuals who have experienced violence or life-threatening situations may develop posttraumatic stress disorder (PTSD). This disorder has the potential to be life-changing and cause negative psychological and medical issues (Rokach, Ahmed, & Patel, 2017). This potentially life-changing nature and consequence of violence affecting women world-wide deserves greater attention to ensure elimination of risk factors, financial support of investigational studies to promote detection of victims, and research to increase therapeutic efficacy of remediation. These efforts should be bolstered by all physicians, mental health experts, social service specialists, and public health advocates.

About one-third of adult females in the United States report experiences of intimate partner violence (IPV). This type of violence may result in posttraumatic stress disorder (PTSD) which is defined in the fifth edition of the Diagnostic and Statistical Manual of Mental Disorders, DSM-5 (APA, 2013) as the posttrauma victim suffering from a constellation of symptoms. The four clusters of symptoms include intrusive and recurrent memories of the trauma, numbing, or negative changes in mood or cognitions related to the trauma, difficulties in reactivity and arousal, and avoidance of trauma-related stimuli. The physical and mental health effects of IPV, risk factors, intervention techniques, and therapeutic options recommended by the American Psychological Association (APA, 2017) will be outlined.

Struggles of Women Victimized by Violence

IPV affects about one-third of women in their lifetimes. This trauma, a type of interpersonal violence, represents a major threat to the physical, mental, or psychological safety and well-being of the victim. This violence results in physiological and psychological stress responses that are overwhelming and challenges the victim's capacity to cope (APA, 2017). A study which was published in 2002 whose authors analyzed data from the National Violence Against Women Survey (NVAWS) of women and men aged 18–65 documented physical IPV victimization was associated with increased risk of poor health, symptoms of depression, substance use, and developing either a chronic mental or physical illness (Coker et al., 2002).

IPV includes sexual coercion, physical aggression, psychological abuse, stalking, and/or controlling behaviors perpetrated by a current or previous intimate partner in a heterosexual or same-sex relationship. This trauma may cause physical injury, increased risk for sexually transmitted diseases, pregnancy complications, and death. Psychological sequelae may include depression, anxiety, PTSD, impulsivity, substance abuse, and suicidality. Victims of IPV may present to healthcare providers with physical signs of trauma, psychological problems as well as nonspecific complaints such as chronic back pain, headaches, generalized fatigue, or weight loss (Stewart, Vigod, & Riazantseva, 2016). Women battered by IPV affected by severe anxiety and depression may use alcohol and drugs excessively. Violence to pregnant women is linked to increased risk for low birth weight infants, preterm delivery, and neonatal death (Sarkar, 2008). In some regions of the world, women exposed to IPV are 1.5 times more likely to acquire HIV and have increased numbers of abortions compared to women who have not been battered (WHO, 2016).

IPV may lead to PTSD causing recurrent dreams or flashbacks of the violent episodes. Individuals with PTSD avoid situations that remind them of the event and often suffer from irritability, hypervigilance, and difficulties with sleep (Stern, Fricchione, Cassem, Jelinek, & Rosenbaum, 2004). When the perpetrator of the assault is a trusted and depended upon individual, the trauma is considered betrayal trauma (Freyd, 1996, p. 76). PTSD has been found to create vulnerability for revictimization (Duckworth & Follette, 2012). It can be potentially life-changing as well as causing threatening psychological and medical issues (Rokach, Ahmed, & Patel, 2017).

The Enormity and Consequences of Violence Against Women

Homicide is one of the leading causes of death for women less than 44 years of age. In 2015, homicide caused the death of 3519 girls and women in the United States with nearly half of the victims killed by a current or former male intimate partner. During 2003–2014 in 18 states over half of all homicides of women 18 years old or greater were related to IPV. In the month prior to the homicides, over 10% of the victims had experienced some form of violence (Petrosky, Blair, Betz, & Fowler, 2017).

The Complex Needs of Women Victimized by Betrayal Trauma

About 30% of the general female adult population report being physically assaulted by a current or former spouse, partner, boyfriend, or date (CDC, 2017a). Most female victims of assault are victims of IPV which affects their psychological and physical health directly by injury and indirectly through a prolonged stress response that leads to chronic health problems. The influence of abuse can cause trauma long after the violence has stopped. The more severe the intimate partner abuse, the greater its impact on health. The longer the abuse continues, the more cumulative the damage to the victim (Dahlberg & Mercy, 2009; Heise & Garcia, 2002).

Those who have been victims of IPV are at great risk of poor health, depression, substance use and chronic mental illness (CDC, 2017a). Domestic violence survivors develop PTSD and depression resulting from feeling a sense of helplessness, ongoing threats to safety and anticipatory fear (Salcioglu et al., 2017). They may also suffer from general anxiety disorder (Cody, Jones, Woodward, Simmons, & Beck, 2015).

Women who are victims of IPV have a three to five times greater likelihood of depression, suicidality, PTSD, and substance abuse than nonvictims. The prevalence rates of PTSD among battered women vary from 31% to 84.4% (Jones, Hughes, & Unterstaller, 2001). In contrast, PTSD affects 3.5% of the adult US population (Bear, Connors, & Paradiso, 2016 p. 757). PTSD is associated with emotional dysregulation including flashbacks, startle responses, hypervigilance as well as emotional shutdown. It may lead to feelings of isolation, changes in cognition and moral questioning (APA, 2017). Victims of PTSD may exhibit risk taking, abuse themselves or others, become addicted to illicit substances and have difficulty with maintaining intimate and trusting relationships. Decreased ability to function at work may lead to job loss, anger, and criminal actions (APA, 2017).

Intimate partner emotional abuse as well as absence of partner caring and respectful behavior may lead to physical and mental health symptoms in addition to diminished quality of life (Queen, Brackley, & Williams, 2009). Women who are in abusive relationships may have feelings of loneliness, isolation, and social marginalization (Rokash, 2007).

Complex PTSD

Victims of chronic trauma that continued for months or years may exhibit additional symptoms alongside those more typical of PTSD. Complex PTSD may develop in women who have been traumatized for years by abusive partners and in persons who suffered years of child physical or sexual abuse. These victims often struggle with poor self-perception with feelings of stigma, seeing themselves as different from other persons, and a sense of helplessness. In addition to the "usual" symptoms of PTSD, victims of chronic trauma may have difficulties with explosive anger, a sense of dissociation, preoccupation with seeking revenge, distrust, and chronic sense of despair. They may engage in self-mutilation, use alcohol or other substances, and have overwhelming feelings associated with the traumatic experiences (Herman, 1997).

Depression as an Independent Risk Factor for Cardiac Disease and a Systemic Illness

Depression is ubiquitous among victims of high betrayal trauma. Depression is additionally an independent risk factor for cardiac disease and is common among victims of childhood abuse and IPV. Women with depression, therefore, need careful evaluation for lipid management, diet, physical activity, and smoking. (Lutwak & Dill, 2012b, 2012c).

Depression is additionally a systemic disease that affects multiple medical illnesses via neurobiological mechanisms (Lutwak & Dill, 2012a, 2012b, 2012c; Sotelo & Nemeroff, 2017). It is a complicating factor of heart disease, stroke, diabetes, osteoporosis, and cancer. Diverse biological processes are influenced by depression and increased levels of proinflammatory cytokines are associated with anxiety. Inflammation, alterations in autonomic nervous system activity, and neuroendocrine dysregulation may, in turn, lead to the progression of depression in the setting of cooccurring medical disease. Experiences of childhood and adult trauma may magnify psychological as well as physiological illness (Sotelo & Nemeroff, 2017). Adulthood medical maladies may be affected by early childhood trauma through mechanisms of increased inflammation and hypothalamic-pituitary-adrenal axis activity (Sotelo & Nemeroff, 2017). Women with histories of childhood maltreatment have higher rates of physical health problems and greater medical utilization compared to women without abuse histories. Women with PTSD as well as depression have more medical conditions and worse physical problems, bodily pain, and lower energy levels than women with depression alone (Frayne et al., 2004; Lang et al., 2006).

Social Challenges of Women Who are Victims of High Betrayal Trauma

Domestic violence is one of the leading causes of homelessness for women and children. Among US city mayors surveyed in 2005, 50% identified IPV as a primary cause of homelessness in their city. Unemployment may also increase risk of homelessness and medical noncompliance (Hamilton, Poza, & Washington, 2011).

Being homeless introduces instability in daily life and may lead to problems for women adhering to scheduled preventive care and compliance with taking medications (Elsevier Health, 2014; Hunter et al., 2014). Smoking rates are high among homeless individuals making chronic obstructive pulmonary disease more likely (Baggett, Lebrun-Harris, & Rigotti, 2013; Baggett, Tobey, & Rigotti, 2013; Tsai & Rosenheck, 2012). People who are homeless are also at increased risk for premature death and contracting tuberculosis (Hwang, 2001). Being homeless is associated with pain and increased visits to emergency rooms (Doran et al., 2014). Thus, IPV resulting in homelessness has multiple psychological as well as medical consequences (Elsevier Health, 2014).

Data from the CDC indicate the pervasiveness of IPV against women in the general population with only about one-third of injured female rape and physical assault victims receiving medical treatment. Clearly violence prevention strategies are needed, there should be better detection of women at risk and public health authorities must encourage women who have been assaulted to seek proper medical care, psychological therapy, and social support (CDC, 2017a).

Risk Factors for IPV, Prevention, and Intervention Strategies

Risk factors may be better understood using the ecological model which organizes the likelihood of IPV into four levels of influence. They include the individual level, which encapsulates biological and personal history factors, the relationship level which includes association with one's closest social circle, community level which includes workplace, schools, and neighborhoods and finally the societal macro level. The latter larger societal level includes cultural belief systems, economic policies, religious beliefs, and issues of gender inequality. Interventions for prevention of IPV may be instituted at all four levels (CDC, 2017b)

Interventions in Schools

Dating violence is widespread, frequently unreported by fearful teens, and the cause of serious long-term and short-term consequences. A 2017 Center for Disease Control report found that approximately 7% of women who ever experienced rape, physical violence, or stalking by an intimate partner first experienced some form of violence by that partner before 18 years of age (CDC, 2017c). Data from high school students who participated in the Maryland Safe and

Supportive Schools Initiative revealed 11% of students experienced physical teen dating violence (TDV) during the year prior to the study, with the same percentage experiencing psychological TDV over the same time period. The study showed alcohol use was associated with teen dating violence. Efforts to reduce teenage alcohol use might reduce TDV and future IPV (Parker, Johnson, Debnam, Milam, & Bradshaw, 2017).

The psychological consequences for young women of experiencing physical teen dating violence are an important factor contributing to future victimization a few years later. This has potential implications for advocating institution school-based programs to eliminate physical teen dating violence. Prevention of teen dating violence may lead to reduced future violence toward women (Jouriles, Choi, Rancher, & Temple, 2017).

Prevention and Detection in Healthcare Settings

Identifying victims of high betrayal trauma in all emergency departments nationally is paramount to enable provision of healing therapy and effective care management (Lutwak, 2014; Lutwak & Dill, 2012d; Lutwak & Dill 2013). The recognition of warning signs of abuse by providers at community health centers is also needed (Women's Health, 2017; HHS, 2017). In 2012, the United States Preventive Services Task Force recommended routine screening of all women of child-bearing age for abuse and IPV. The American College of Emergency Physicians subsequently issued a policy that such screening should be performed in emergency department settings. Screening for IPV is also recommended by the National Center of Injury Prevention and Control, as well as the American Medical Association. Screening for IPV has been instituted at Veteran Health Administration emergency departments nationally, given the scope and negative consequences of this problem (Lutwak, 2014).

Lack of privacy, lack of time, work pressure, inappropriate environment, poor knowledge of protocols, unwillingness of healthcare professionals, unclear referral pathways, lack of professional involvement in policies, and unclear prompts may decrease detection rates. Inattentiveness of professionals, lack of empathy, inappropriate training to develop confidence in asking sensitive questions and gender incongruence of screeners all play a part in poor detection of victimization. More effective screening must be in place since IPV detection is essential to help prevent further victimization (Ahmad, Ali, Rehman, Talpur, & Dhingra, 2017). Better provider patient communication about IPV is required (Rhodes et al., 2007). Verbal-based screening can be effective when the practitioner is skilled at developing rapport and trust. Use of computer-based detection is effective since the victim may answer questions without being interrupted, without embarrassment or feeling they are being judged. Culturally specific tools for different populations may be needed (Ahmad et al., 2017).

Women in chronic relationships who are battered may seek help in acute care settings more than once. Greatest risk factors for escalation of violence are linked to victim's age greater than 20, children present in the home and the perpetrator reported as dating partner or ex-partner (Brignone & Gomez, 2017). Contacting social service support services to alert them of women screening positive for IPV or those with frequent visits to emergency departments with possible symptoms related to being battered is requisite. Tools may include use of e-messaging in healthcare settings for immediate consultations and telehealth to contact patients in need of rapid support (Brignone & Gomez, 2017).

Interventions to Prevent and Treat Homelessness, Substance Abuse, Pain, and Suicidality

Suicide remains a major public health concern as the tenth leading cause of adult deaths in the United States (Hoffberg, Spitzer, Mackelprang, Farro, & Brenner, 2017). Prevalence of suicidal ideation and suicidal attempts among homeless adults is higher compared to a recent national sample of adults (Dietz, 2010). Homelessness and domestic violence for women and children overlap necessitating greater advocacy for the victims and funding from the U.S. Department of Housing and Urban Development for shelters and temporary domiciles (Department of Housing, 2018).

Women with substance use disorders have increased risk of suicide (Bohnert, Ilgen, Louzon, McCarthy, & Katz, 2017). Proinflammatory cytokines are now known to oppose opioid-induced acute and chronic analgesia suggesting that heightened depression or anxiety leads to increased production of interleukin-1 (Hutchinson et al., 2008). That might decrease the effectiveness of opioids resulting in need for increased doses and greater chance of addiction (Hutchinson et al., 2008; Olsen, Rollins, & Billhard, 2013).

Since depression affects severity of chronic pain the urgency of mental health treatment is magnified as is the importance of more effective strategies of pain management. Use of non-addictive medication with concurrent holistic approaches including acupuncture, physical therapy, mind-body medicine, diet, and exercise/movement protocols should be considered (Hillinger, Wolever, McKernan, & Elam, 2017; Sehgal, Manchikanti, & Smith, 2012).

Healthcare providers should focus on the complex interplay between medical illness, psychological distress, trauma, suicidal ideation, and social problems. Routine screening for depression in all age groups and gender is requisite in all medical facilities since this disorder acts as a mediator leading to deterioration of medical diseases. The bidirectional interaction of depression and cardiovascular disease, cancer, renal disease, stroke, and diabetes should additionally be incorporated into healthcare decisions. This is important in rendering excellent care for women many of whom have experienced abuse in childhood and adulthood. Detection of IPV which leads to depression, chronic pain, suicidal ideation, PTSD, and medical illness (Sotelo & Nemeroff, 2017) is essential.

Strategies to Heal the Wounds of High Betrayal Trauma

Betrayal trauma is a type of trauma that involves violation by a person one trusts for survival or well-being (Freyd, 1996, p. 76). Child abuse and IPV are examples of betrayal trauma which may result in complex PTSD with feelings of negative self-perception, hopelessness, difficulty trusting others, shame, guilt, and impulsivity (McLean & Follette, 2016; Olsen et al., 2013). Depression as well as somatic problems result and victims may require comprehensive care for recovery including medical/psychiatric/social help in addition to legal advocacy services, support with child care, employment assistance as well as housing/economic help (Women's Health, 2017; HHS, 2017).

Childhood abuse and IPV leave painful deep scars, feelings of shame and guilt, anger, depression, fear, and lack of self-acceptance. Recovery may take years but multiple strategies are available to heal the wounds. Trauma exposure may lead to persistent symptomatology, however, the manner in which the victims think about and assess their experiences are important in determining the length and severity of distress. The quantity of traumas experienced and the relationship of the victim to the perpetrator are meaningful, but the appraisal of the trauma by the victim may be more significant in affecting the long-term impact (Martin, Cromer, DePrince, & Freyd, 2013).

Identification of victims and providing safe havens is an important step in recovery. Social support from trusted family members, friends, religious leaders, doctors, or nurses resulting in feelings of connection is another helpful strategy to start recovery (DVA, 2017a).

PTSD, depression, alcohol, and substance abuse are among the mental health effects of traumatization. PTSD may lead to personality-based vulnerability to responding negatively in the context of distress. Aggressive risk taking behavior resulting in negative consequences for individuals suffering from PTSD may be modified by psychological flexibility. Learning the skill of flexibility enables those with PTSD to make decisions consistent with positive goals even during stress, thereby avoiding negative urgency (Dutra & Sadeh, 2017).

PTSD and substance use disorder commonly occur together leading to impairment of functioning (Mason, Wolf, O'Rinn, & Ene, 2017). Individual-based trauma-focused cognitive behavioral therapy plus concurrent adjunctive substance use disorder intervention reduce levels of distress (Roberts, Roberts, Jones, & Bisson, 2016). Coordinated treatment between mental health providers, therapists to treat substance abuse and primary care doctors is essential (Mason et al., 2017). The team of providers must be cognizant that the stress of abuse may result in depression, anxiety, overeating, hypertension, and headaches. It may also increase risk of heart disease, stroke, and lead to poor medical compliance worsening chronic illness such as diabetes (Sotelo & Nemeroff, 2017). The importance of a team approach to improve care of battered women and those who experienced childhood assault is paramount (Machisa, Christofides, & Jewkes, 2017).

Complex Care Management Programs

Trauma and chronic stress lead to poor psychological and physical health. Approximately 22%–30% of women experience physical, sexual, or psychological IPV during their lifetime (Women's Health, 2017; HHS, 2017). Poor healthcare outcomes occur as patients often experience fragmented, bureaucratic systems which are difficult to navigate. Complex care management programs utilizing interdisciplinary teams of providers to promote healing using trauma informed primary care are effective. These programs employ coordinated medical, behavioral health, and social service providers working together to improve chronic illness, access to food, housing, transportation, and engagement from family members. The team of physicians, nurses, social workers, and community outreach workers cooperate to increase medical adherence, reduce substance abuse, secure housing, and support self-management of chronic medical conditions (Thompson-Lastad et al., 2017).

Skillsets to Help Cope with Trauma and Alleviate Distress

Personal growth initiative (PGI), a skillset for promoting change in one's self through focus on developing realistic plans with use of available resources and accomplishing the envisioned action plan, may be useful to adapt after traumatic events. Persons with high intent of personal growth may have less distress following a traumatic event and greater ability to cope.

People with greater self-esteem may benefit from making decisions and thinking positively of future plans while engaging actively in making life changes. Avoiding unproductive rumination and developing high personal mastery may increase posttraumatic growth. Reflective coping strategies, acting on personal growth and productive thinking may protect against depression. People with commitment, control, and psychological hardiness may experience less stress posttrauma (Shigemoto, Low, Borowa, & Robitschek, 2017). Deliberate rumination and the cognitive component of PGI negatively predicts posttraumatic stress (Shigemoto, Ashton, & Robitschek, 2015).

Current Evidence-based Interventions and Some under Investigation

The American Psychological Association has published recommendation guidelines regarding PTSD treatment based on symptom reduction, improvement in quality of life, prevention or reduction of comorbid medical or psychiatric conditions, and functional impairment. Their strong recommendations include cognitive behavioral therapy, cognitive processing therapy, cognitive therapy, and prolonged exposure therapy. The guidelines do not recommend psychotherapy before or instead of medications (APA, 2017).

Cognitive processing therapy is effective for treating PTSD and depression, however, for increased success, therapists must have good treatment fidelity (Holder, Holliday, Williams, Mullen, & Suris, 2017). Two additional evidence-based interventions include cognitive trauma therapy for battered women and helping to overcome PTSD through empowerment. Cognitive trauma therapy for battered women emphasizes the role of irrational beliefs and evaluative language in chronic PTSD. It includes trauma history exploration, PTSD psychoeducation, and stress management. Helping to overcome PTSD through empowerment targets maladaptive cognitions about self, others, and the world with additional focus on increasing individual safety, sense of control/power/self-esteem, and ability to establish intimate relationships (Gerber et al., 2014).

Acceptance and commitment therapy fosters psychological flexibility aimed at improving adaptation to life's demands and focusing on personal goals. Depression is improved with acceptance of feelings and memories rather than through control of thoughts with avoidance of internal experiences. This technique does not focus on evaluation of symptoms but rather on creation of satisfying, fulfilling lives. This approach supports health with emphasis on living in the present moment. It guides trauma victims in moving forward with life while accepting previous traumatic events. The therapy reinforces the concept that despite negative experiences, it is possible to have a full and meaningful life. Survivors of trauma are helped by embracing the present and not being entrenched in old unpleasant memories. The aim is to find a positive sense of self and feel valuable despite having had painful experiences. The traumatic events are not denied but the aim is to avoid those experiences from defining one's current life (McLean & Follette, 2016; Schnurr & Lunney, 2016).

Present centered therapy, another useful innovative technique, is client-directed problem solving. It focuses on current life concerns and the connection between those concerns and the individual's symptoms (Schnurr & Lunney, 2016).

Use of telemedicine has shown promise for treatment of PTSD. Although there are multiple effective therapies for PTSD, geographic barriers impede rural patients from engaging in these evidence-based treatments. Telemedicine-based collaborative care is effective in treatment of PTSD and is useful to help patients in isolated areas. This technique utilizes off-site

PTSD care teams consisting of telephone nurse care managers, telephone pharmacists, telepsychologists, and telepsychiatrists located at Veteran Health Administration medical centers supported by on-site community-based outpatient clinic providers. Nurses conduct care management activities, pharmacists review medication histories, and psychologists deliver cognitive processing therapy via interactive video. The teams are supervised by psychiatrists who also conduct interactive video psychiatric consultations. Previous evaluation of the effectiveness of such telemedicine techniques measured medication prescribing, regimen adherence and initiation of and adherence to cognitive processing therapy. Patients receiving the telemedicine outreach approach had significantly larger decreases in Posttraumatic Diagnostic Scale scores compared to their counterparts who had usual treatment. In that study, attendance at eight or more sessions of cognitive processing therapy significantly predicted improvement in Posttraumatic Diagnostic Scale scores. Telemedicine-based collaborative care can successfully render evidence-based psychotherapy to improve PTSD outcomes (Fortney et al., 2015).

Therapy for complex PTSD includes usual evidence-based treatment for PTSD, but it may involve addressing interpersonal difficulties as well as restoring feelings of control, safety, power while reconnecting with everyday life (Herman, 1997).

Medication for PTSD

Biological Disturbance in PTSD, Anxiety Disorders

PTSD may cause flashbacks, traumatic memories, self-blame, sleep problems, and anger. Cognitive behavioral therapy as well as psychopharmacology may be quite effective in the road to recovery. Experiences of IPV and child abuse result in enormous traumatic stress (Olsen et al., 2013) with severe mental health and physical debilities (Women's Health, 2017; HHS, 2017). Biological disequilibrium may result (Bear et al., 2016).

The biological disturbance causing PTSD involves dysregulation of the hypothalamic-pituitary-adrenal axis leading to hyperarousal. In PTSD, amygdala activation is adversely affected. Patients with PTSD have increased activation of the amygdala when they perceive stimuli as threatening (Bear et al., 2016). This activation influences the hippocampus, the orbital frontal cortex, the locus coeruleus, thalamus, hypothalamus as well as the dorsal/ventral striatum. The decreased restraints on amygdala activation, particularly on the anterior cingulate gyrus and orbitofrontal cortex, cause inaccurate appraisal of stimuli as threatening. This also results in sensitization of key limbic nuclei thereby lowering the threshold for fearful reactivity (DVA, 2017a).

Anxiety reactions additionally occur with hyperactivity of the amygdala, and diminished activity of the hippocampus after reception of information from the prefrontal cortex. The goal of psychotherapy is to increase exposure of the patient to stimuli that frequently produce anxiety to reinforce the idea that those stimuli are not dangerous. The goal is to alter connections of the brain so that the stimuli that produce fear no longer evoke the stress reaction. Medications which regulate the amygdala which increases the stress response and the hippocampus which suppresses it may be essential in addition to therapy in some cases (Bear et al., 2016).

GABA, gamma-aminobutyric acid, which is an inhibitory neurotransmitter of the brain also plays a part in anxiety disorders. The active ingredient in alcohol stimulates actions of

GABA leading to decreased anxiety. Medications that stimulate GABA actions, such as the benzodiazepines, are also anxiolytic. This explains the frequent use of alcohol and misuse of benzodiazepines by individuals with anxiety disorder or PTSD (Bear et al., 2016).

Medications which improve the symptomatology of depression and anxiety modulate serotonin, norepinephrine, gamma-aminobutyric acid, N-methyl-D-aspartate, and dopamine levels. The FDA has approved the selective serotonin reuptake inhibitors (SSRIs) sertraline and paroxetine for treatment of PTSD. Veteran Health Administration clinical practice guidelines additionally include use of the SSRIs fluoxetine, paroxetine and the serotonin and norepinephrine reuptake inhibitor venlafaxine. Mirtazapine added to sertraline may be helpful as well. Benzodiazepines worsen symptom outcomes in patients with PTSD, are addictive and are not recommended for long-term use (DVA, 2017a).

Second-line medications for PTSD include nefazodone, imipramine, and phenelzine. Topiramate is additionally an option for those who did not respond to first-line therapies (DVA, 2017a), but the American Psychological Association guidelines indicate insufficient evidence to recommend it (APA, 2017).

For women with major depressive disorder (MDD) who do not respond adequately to standard treatments, augmentation of conventional antidepressants with creatine monohydrate and 5-hydroxytryptophan (5-HTP) holds promise. Deficits in serotonin production and brain bioenergetics is associated with depression in women. There may be a synergistic benefit of addition of 5-HTP and creatine augmentation in women with MDD who previously failed selective serotonin reuptake inhibitor (SSRI) or serotonin-norepinephrine reuptake inhibitor (SNRI) monotherapy. Women who have SSRI- or SNRI-resistant depression may improve with this augmentation approach (Kious, Sabic, Sung, Kondo, & Renshaw, 2017).

Medications Posttrauma Exposure

Acute interventions with corticotropin releasing factor antagonists or glucocorticoids following trauma exposure may reduce excessive stress-induced hypothalamus-pituitary-adrenal activation which may have neurotoxic effects. Pharmacological intervention for acute posttraumatic reactions includes targeting the adrenergic system to inhibit excessive alpha-1 and beta receptor activation and to increase inhibition of alpha-2 adrenergic receptors. This downregulates amygdala activity with decreased stimulation of secondary cortical and subcortical structures (DVA, 2017a).

Neurotoxicity may play a role in PTSD. Certain anticonvulsants, which block excitatory amino acid actions and prevent toxic calcium influx decrease neurotoxicity. The SSRI paroxetine also reverses neurotoxicity by promoting neurogenesis and increasing hippocampal volume which may be useful in treatment of PTSD (DVA, 2017a).

PTSD and Substance use Disorder (SUD)

Adherence to addiction-focused pharmacotherapy is recommended. Naltrexone and disulfiram should be offered as a treatment strategy for alcohol use disorder as they may have some direct benefit for PTSD symptoms. Buprenorphine/naloxone might be useful and benzodiazepines alleviate alcohol withdrawal but after detoxification are not recommended for chronic use (DVA, 2017b).

Sertraline and paroxetine have FDA approval as first-line recommended treatments in PTSD. They may be considered for PTSD with or without cooccurring SUD. Use of

additional medications may be prescribed for those with concurrent SUD after consulting with pharmacotherapy specialists (DVA, 2017b).

Conclusion

The prevalence of violence against girls and women in our society is alarming. The immediate and future consequences are dire necessitating greater focus on prevention and effective treatment. Childhood abuse and IPV are forms of high betrayal trauma creating severe and long-lasting negative consequences. Survivors may require support from medical, mental health, and social service experts to improve quality of life, reduce depression, decrease stress, ameliorate physical symptoms, and prevent suicidal ideology. There may be need for economic and employment assistance as well as placement in safe housing. Institutional-based strategies to reduce teen dating violence and alcohol use may diminish trauma in future years. Identification of the victims in all medical and psychological treatment centers is paramount to prevent recurrence of abuse and to offer multiple complex therapies to help heal the deep scars. Chronic pain, substance abuse, and social isolation may worsen the initial posttraumatic ill effects.

Despite the severe trauma, recovery is possible through psychological interventions, pharmacotherapy, and supportive networks. The trauma informed team approach is effective for ameliorating the shame, guilt, anger, depression, and somatic manifestations of the victimization. Several innovative types of therapy are effective and should be offered after evaluating each victim's psychological stage and resilience. Presenting mental health treatment options with or without medication is imperative to ensure compliance and increased success. Learning skillsets of PGI may be useful to reduce stress. The significance of depression as an independent risk factor for cardiac disease, its influence on diverse biological processes and complicating factor of stroke, diabetes, osteoporosis, and cancer require attention by healthcare providers. An integrated team approach for improvement of psychological problems, physical illness, and social issues such as alcohol and drug dependency is needed to hasten recovery from betrayal trauma. Connection to friends, trusted family, other trauma survivors as well as clergy also diminish the sense of isolation to aid in the road to recovery. Finally, prevention and intervention strategies in school settings, the workplace, neighborhoods, and society as a whole should be instituted to promote gender equality and negate the acceptability of violence against women.

References

Ahmad, I., Ali, P. A., Rehman, S., Talpur, A., & Dhingra, K. (2017). Intimate partner violence screening in emergency department: A rapid review of the literature. *Journal of Clinical Nursing*, *26*(21-22), 3271–3285. doi:10.1111/jocn.13706

APA. (2013). *Diagnostic and statistical manual of mental disorders: DSM-5*. Washington DC: American Psychiatric Association.

APA. (2017). PTSD Guidelines. https://www.apa.org/ptsd-guideline/ptsd.pdf

Baggett, T. P., Tobey, M. L., & Rigotti, N. A. (2013). Tobacco use among homeless people—Addressing the neglected addiction. *New England Journal of Medicine, 369*(3), 201–204. doi:10.1056/NEJMp1301935

Baggett, T. P., Lebrun-Harris, L. A., & Rigotti, N. A. (2013). Homelessness, cigarette smoking and desire to quit: Results from a US national study. *Addiction, 108*(11), 2009–2018. doi:10.1111/add.12292

Bear, M. F., Connors, B. W., & Paradiso, M. A. (2016). *Neuroscience exploring the brain* (4th ed., pp. 754–763). New York, NY: Wolters Kluwer.

Bohnert K. M., Ilgen, M. A., Louzon, S., McCarthy, J. F., & Katz, I. R. (2017). Substance use disorders and the risk of suicide mortality among men and women in the US Veterans Health Administration. *Addiction, 112*(7):1193–1201. doi:10.1111/add.13774

Brignone, L., & Gomez, A. M. (2017). Double jeopardy: Predictors of elevated lethality risk among intimate partner violence victims seen in emergency departments. *Preventive Medicine, 103*, 20–25. [Epub ahead of print] CDC.gov/violenceprevention/intimatepartnerviolence/datasources.html Data sources available at https://www.cdc.gov doi:10.1016/j.ypmed.2017.06.035

CDC. (2017a). Intimate partner violence. Accessed 06 April, 2018 from https://www.cdc.gov/violence prevention/intimatepartnerviolence/index.html

CDC. (2017b). Prevent domestic violence in your community. Accessed 06 April, 2018 from https://www.cdc.gov/features/intimatepartnerviolence/index.html

CDC. (2017c). Intimate partner violence: Data sources. Accessed 02 February, 2017 from https://www.cdc.gov/violenceprevention/intimatepartnerviolence/datasources.html

Cody, M. W., Jones, J. M., Woodward, M. J., Simmons, C. A., & Beck, J. G. (2015). Correspondence between self-report measures and clinician assessments of psychopathology in female intimate partner violence survivors. *Journal of Interpersonal Violence, 32*, 1501–1523. doi:10.1177/0886260515589566

Coker, A. L., Davis, K. E., Arias, I., Desai, S., Sanderson, M., Brandt, H. M., & Smith, P. H. (2002). Physical and mental health effects of intimate partner violence for men and women. *American Journal of Preventive Medicine, 23*, 260–268. doi:10.1016/S0749-3797(02)00514-7

Dahlberg, L. L., & Mercy, J. A. (2009). History of violence as a public health issue. *Virtual Mentor, 11*, 167–172. doi:10.1001/virtualmentor.2009.11.2.mhst1-0902

Dardis, C. M., Amoroso, T., & Iverson, K. M. (2017). Intimate partner stalking: Contributions to PTSD symptomatology among a national sample of women veterans. *Psychological Trauma, 9* (Suppl 1), 67–73. Epub 2016 Jul 14. Department of Defense, Psychological Health Webinars, available at dcoe@service.govdelivery.com doi:10.1037/tra0000171

Department of Housing. (2018). Domestic Violence and Homelessness: HUD exchange. Accessed 06 April 2018 from https://www.hudexchange.info/homelessness-assistance/domestic-violence

Dichter, M. E., Haywood, T. N., Butler, A. E., Bellamy, S. L., & Iverson, K. M. (2017). Intimate partner violence screening in the veterans health administration: Demographic and military service characteristics. *American Journal of Preventive Medicine, 52*(6), 761–768. doi:10.1016/j.amepre.2017.01.003

Dietz, T. L. (2010) Substance Misuse, Suicidal Ideation and Suicide Attempts Among a National Sample of Homeless. *Journal of Social Service*, 37, 1–18.

Doran, K. M., Shumway, M., Hoff, R. A., Blackstock, O. J., Dilworth, S. E., & Riley, E. D. (2014). Correlates of hospital use in homeless and unstably housed women: The role of physical health and pain. *Women's Health Issues : Official Publication of the Jacobs Institute of Women's Health, 24*, 535–541. doi:10.1016/j.whi.2014.06.003

Duckworth, M. P., & Follette, V. M. (2012). *Retraumatization: Assessment, treatment, and prevention.* New York: Routledge Taylor and Francis Group.

Dutra, S. J., & Sadeh, M. (2017). Psychological flexibility mitigates effects of PTSD symptoms and negative urgency on aggressive behavior in trauma-exposed veterans. *Personality Disorders: Theory, Research, and Treatment.* doi:10.1037/per0000251

DVA. (2017a). Treatment of Co-Occurring PTSD and Substance Use Disorder in VA. https://www.ptsd.va.gov/professional/co-occurring/ptsd_sud_veterans.asp

DVA. (2017b). Treatment of PTSD—PTSD: National Center for PTSD. https://www.ptsd.va.gov/public/treatment/therapy-med/treatment-ptsd.asp

Elsevier Health. (2014). Noncompliance. Available at www1.us.elsevierhealth.com/MERLIN/Gulanick/.../gulanick35.html

Fortney, J. C., Pyne, J. M., Kimbrell, T. A., Hudson, T. J., Robinson, D. E., Schneider, R., Moore, W. M., Custer, P. J., Grubbs, K. M., & Schnurr, P. P. (2015). Telemedicine-based collaborative care for posttraumatic stress disorder: A randomized clinical trial. *JAMA Psychiatry, 72*, 58–67. doi:10.1001/jamapsychiatry.2014.1575

Frayne, S. M., Seaver, M. R., Loveland, S., Christiansen, C. L., Spiro, A., Parker, V. A., & Skinner, K. (2004). Burden of medical illness in women with depression and posttraumatic stress disorder. *Archives of Internal Medicine, 164*(12), 1306–1312. doi:10.1001/archinte.164.12.1306

Freyd, J. J. (1996). *Betrayal trauma: The Logic of forgetting childhood abuse*. Harvard University Press.

Gerber, M. R., Iverson, K. M., Dichter, M. E., Klap, R., & Latta, R. E. (2014) Women veterans and intimate partner violence: Current state of knowledge and future directions. *Journal of Women's Health, 23*(4), 302–309.

Hamilton, A. B., Poza, I., & Washington, D. L. (2011). Homelessness and trauma go hand-in-hand: Pathways to homelessness among women veterans. *Women's Health Issues, 21*(4 Suppl), S203–S209. doi:10.1016/j.whi.2011.04.005

Heise, L., & Garcia, M. C. (2002). Violence by intimate partners. In Krug EG (Ed.), *World report on violence and health* (pp. 87–121). Geneva, Switzerland: World Health Organization.

Herman, J. (1997). Trauma and recovery: The aftermath of violence from domestic abuse to political terror. New York, NY: Basic Books.

HHS. (2017). Safety from violence & abuse. Accessed 07 April, 2018 from https://www.hhs.gov/programs/public-health-safety/safety-from-violence-abuse/index.html

Hoffberg, A. S., Spitzer, E., Mackelprang, J. L., Farro, S. A., & Brenner, L. A. (2017). Suicidal self-directed violence among homeless US veterans: A systematic review. *Suicide and Life-Threatening Behavior*, 2017 Jul 21. doi:10.1111/sltb.12369

Holder, N., Holliday, R., Williams, R., Mullen, K., & Suris, A. (2017). A preliminary examination of the role of psychotherapist fidelity on outcomes of cognitive processing therapy during an RCT for military sexual-trauma-related PTSD. *Cognitive Behavioural Therapy, 10*, 1–14. doi:10.1080/16506073.2017.1357750.

Hillinger, M. G., Wolever, R. Q., McKernan, L. C., & Elam, R. (2017). Integrative medicine for the treatment of persistent pain. *Primary Care, 44*(2), 247–264. doi:10.1016/j.pop.2017.02.008

Hutchinson, M. R., Coats, B. D., Lewis, S. S., Zhang, Y., Sprunger, D. B., & Rezvani, N. (2008).et al. Proinflammatory cytokines oppose opioid induced acute and chronic analgesia. *Brain, Behavior, and Immunity, 22*(8), 1178–1189. doi:10.1016/j.bbi.2008.05.004

Hunter, C. E., Palepu, A., Farrell, S., Gogosis, E., O'Brien, K., & Hwang, S. W. (2014). Barriers to prescription medication adherence among homeless and vulnerably housed adults in three Canadian cities. *Journal of Primary Care & Community Health, 6*(3), 154–161.

Hwang, S. W. (2001). Homelessness and health. *Canadian Medical Association Journal, 164*, 229–233.

Jones, L., Hughes, M., & Unterstaller, U. (2001). Post-traumatic stress disorder (PTSD) in victims of domestic violence: A review of the research. *Trauma, Violence, & Abuse, 2*, 99–119. doi:10.1177/1524838001002002001

Jouriles, E. N., Choi, H. J., Rancher, C., & Temple, J. R. (2017). Teen dating violence victimization, trauma symptoms, and revictimization in early adulthood. *Journal of Adolescent Health, 61*(1), 115–119. Epub 2017 Mar 28. doi:10.1016/j.jadohealth.2017.01.020

Kious, B. M., Sabic, H., Sung, Y. H., Kondo, D. G., & Renshaw, P. (2017). An open-label pilot study of combined augmentation with creatine monohydrate and 5-hydroxytryptophan for selective serotonin reuptake inhibitor- or serotonin-norepinephrine reuptake inhibitor-resistant depression in adult women. *Journal of Clinical Psychopharmacology, 37*(5), 578–583. [Epub ahead of print] doi:10.1097/JCP.0000000000000754

Lang, A. J., Laffaye, C., Satz, L. E., McQuaid, J. R., Malcarne, V. L., Dresselhaus, T. R., & Stein, M. B. (2006). Relationships among childhood maltreatment, PTSD, and health in female veterans in primary care. *Child Abuse and Neglect, 30*(11), 1281–1292. doi:10.1016/j.chiabu.2006.06.005

Lang, A. J., Schnurr, P. P., Jain, S., He, F., Walser, R. D., Bolton, E., & Benedek, D. M. (2016). Randomized Controlled Trial of Acceptance and Commitment Therapy for Distress and Impairment in

OEF/OIF/OND Veterans. Psychological Trauma: Theory Research, Practice and Policy. June 2016. doi:10.1037/tra0000127

Lindsay, J. A., Kauth, M. R., & Hudson, S. (2015). Implementation of video telehealth to improve access to evidence-based psychotherapy for posttraumatic stress disorder. *Telemedicine Journal and e-Health, 21*(6), 467–472. doi:10.1089/tmj.2014.0114

Lutwak, N. (2014). Screening for intimate partner violence at VA EDs: The time is now. *Journal of General Internal Medicine, 29*(2), 279. doi:10.1007/s11606-013-2717-5

Lutwak, N., & Dill, C. (2012a). The mind body connection and cardiovascular disease. International *Journal of Clinical Practice, 66*(11), 1126–1127. doi:10.1111/ijcp.12002

Lutwak, N., & Dill, C. (2012b). Depression and cardiovascular disease in women. *Journal of Women's Health, 21*(6), 702. author reply 703. Epub 2012 Apr 20. doi:10.1089/jwh.2012.3626

Lutwak, N., & Dill, C. (2012c). A depressed post-menopausal woman. *Journal of Emergency Medicine, 43*(5), 815–819. doi:10.1016/j.jemermed.2011.05.040

Lutwak, N., & Dill, C. (2012d). The importance of screening and treating depression in all women. *Journal of Women's Health*, 21(12), 1302. doi:10.1089/jwh.2012.4042

Lutwak, N., Dill, C. (2013) Military sexual trauma increases risk of post-traumatic stress disorder and depression thereby amplifying the possibility of suicidal ideation and cardiovascular disease. *Military Medicine, 178*(4), 359–361. doi:10.7205/MILMED-D-12-00427

Martin, C. G., Cromer, L. D., DePrince, A. P., & Freyd, J. J. (2013). The role of cumulative trauma, betrayal, and appraisals in understanding trauma symptomatology. *Psychological Trauma, 52*(2), 110–118. doi:10.1037/a0025686

McLean, C., & Follette, V. M. (2016). Acceptance and commitment therapy as a nonpathologizing intervention approach for survivors of trauma. *Journal of Trauma & Dissociation, 17*, 138–150. doi:10.1080/15299732.2016.1103111

Mason, R., Wolf, M., O'Rinn, S., & Ene, G. (2017). Making connections across silos: Intimate partner violence, mental health, and substance use. *BMC Women's Health, 17*, 29 doi:10.1186/s12905-017-0372-4

Machisa, M. T., Christofides, N., & Jewkes, R. (2017). Mental ill health in structural pathways to women's experiences of intimate partner violence. *Plos One, 12*(4), e0175240. doi:10.1371/journal.pone.0175240

Montgomery, A. E., Dichter, M. E., Thomasson, A. M., Fu, X., & Roberts, C. B. (2015). Demographic characteristics associated with homelessness and risk among female and male veterans accessing VHA outpatient care. *Womens Health Issues, 25*(1), 42–48. doi:10.1016/j.whi.2014.10.003

Olsen, L., Rollins, C., & Billhard, K. (2013). Domestic Violence Housing First. The Intersection of Domestic Violence and Homelessness. Washington State Coalition Against Domestic Violence.

Parker, E. M., Johnson, S. L., Debnam, K. J., Milam, A. J., & Bradshaw, C. P. (2017). Teen dating violence victimization among high school students: A multilevel analysis of school-level risk factors. *Journal of School Health, 87*(9), 696–704. doi:10.1111/josh.12538

Petrosky, E., Blair, J. M., Betz, C. J., & Fowler, K. A. (2017). Racial and ethnic differences in homicides of adult women and the role of intimate partner violence—United States, 2003–2014. *MMWR Morbidity Mortality Weekly Report, 66*(28), 741–746. doi:10.15585/mmwr.mm6628a1

Queen, J., Brackley, M. H., & Williams, G. B. (2009). Being emotionally abused: A phenomenological study of adult women's experiences of emotionally abusive intimate partner relationships. *Issues in Mental Health Nursing, 30*, 237–245. doi:10.1080/01612840802701257

Rhodes, K. V., Frankel, R. M., Levinthal, N., Prenoveau, E., Bailey, J., & Levinson, W. (2007). "You're not a victim of domestic violence, are you?" Provider patient communication about domestic violence. *Annals of Internal Medicine. 147*(9), 62–27. doi:10.7326/0003-4819-147-9-200711060-00006

Roberts, N. P., Roberts, P. A., Jones, N., & Bisson, J. I. (2016). Psychological therapies for post-traumatic stress disorder and comorbid use disorder. *The Cochrane Library, 4*, CD010204. doi:10.1002/14651858.CD010204

Rokash, A. (2007). Loneliness and intimate partner violence: Antecedents of alienation of abused women. *Social Work Health Care, 45*, 19–31 doi:10.1300/J010v45n01_02

Rokach, A., Ahmed, R., & Patel, K. (2017). Senseless violence: A global problem with psychological ramifications. *Journal of Psychology, 151*(1), 1–4.

Salcioglu, E., Urhan, S., Pirinccioglu, T., & Aydin, S. (2017). Anticipatory fear and helplessness predict PTSD and depression in domestic violence survivors. *Psychological Trauma: Theory, Research, Practice, and Policy, 9*(1), 117–125. doi:10.1037/tra0000200

Sambamoorthi, U., Bean-Mayberry, B., Findley, P. A., Yano, E. M., & Banerjea, R. (2010). Organization of care and diagnosed depression among women veterans. *American Journal of Managed Care, 16*(9), 657–665.

Sarkar, N. N. (2008). The impact of intimate partner violence on women's reproductive health and pregnancy outcome. *Journal of Obstetrics and Gynaecology. 28*(3), 266–271. doi:10.1080/01443610802042415

Schnurr, P. P., & Lunney, C. A. (2016). Symptom benchmarks of improved quality of life in PTSD. *Depression and Anxiety, 33*, 247–255. doi:10.1002/da.22477

Sehgal, N., Manchikanti, L., & Smith, H. S. (2012). Prescription opioid abuse in chronic pain: A review of opioid abuse predictors and strategies to curb opioid abuse. *Pain Physician, 15*(3 Suppl), ES67–ES92.

Shigemoto, Y., Low, B., Borowa, D., & Robitschek, C. (2017). Function of personal growth initiative on posttraumatic growth, posttraumatic stress, and depression over and above adaptive and maladaptive rumination. *Journal of Clinical Psychology, 73*, 1126–1145. doi:10.1002/jclp.22423

Shigemoto, Y., Ashton, M. W., & Robitschek, C. (2015). Predictors of growth in the aftermath of traumatic events: The role of personal growth initiatives, *Journal of Loss and Trauma, 21*, 399–409. doi:10.1080/15325024.2015.1110446

Sotelo, J. L., & Nemeroff, C. B. (2017). Depression as a systemic disease. *Personalized Medicine in Psychiatry, 1–2*, 11–25. doi:10.1016/j.pmip.2016.11.002

Stern, T. A., Fricchione, G. L., Cassem, N. H., Jelinek, M. S., & Rosenbaum, J. F. (2004). *Massachusetts general hospital handbook of general hospital psychiatry* (5th ed., pp. 180–181). Philadelphia: Mosby.

Stewart, D. E., Vigod, S., & Riazantseva, E. (2016). New developments in intimate partner violence and management of its mental health sequelae. *Current Psychiatry Reports, 18*(1), 4. doi:10.1007/s11920-015-0644-3

Thompson-Lastad, A., Yen, I. H., Fleming, M. D., Van Natta, M., Rubin, S., Shim, J. K., & Burke, N. J. (2017). Defining trauma in complex care management: Safety-net providers' perspectives on structural vulnerability and time. *Social Science & Medicine, 186*, 104–112. doi:10.1016/j.socscimed.2017.06.003

Tsai, J., & Rosenheck, R. A. (2012). Smoking among chronically homeless adults: Prevalence and correlates. *Psychiatric Services, 63*, 569–576. doi:10.1176/appi.ps.201100398

Tsai, J., Hoff, R. A., & Harpaz-Rotem, I. (2017). One-year incidence and predictors of homelessness among 300,000 U.S. veterans seen in specialty mental health care. *Psychological Services, 14*(2), 203–207. doi:10.1037/ser0000083

Warner, C., Sewali, B., Olayinka, A., Eischen, S., Wang, Q., Guo, H., Ahluwalia, J. S., & Okuyemi, K. S. (2014). Smoking cessation in homeless populations: Who participates and who does not. *Nicotine & Tobacco Research, 16*(3), 369–372. doi:10.1093/ntr/ntt169

Women's Health. (2017). Domestic or intimate partner violence. Accessed 06 April, 2018 from https://www.womenshealth.gov/relationships-and-safety/domestic-violence

WHO. (2016). Violence against women. www.who.int/mediacentre/factsheets/fs239/en/

Emotion Regulation Difficulties Mediate the Relationship between Neuroticism and Health-Risk Behaviours in Adolescents

Parwinder Singh

ABSTRACT

Health-Risk-Behaviors (HRBs) are significant antecedent conditions of adolescents' poor health and mortality. Prevention of avoidable adverse health outcomes requires an in-depth understanding of the factors associated with such outcomes. Among other possible pathways, the 'Neuroticism- HRBs-adverse health' link has been supported in previous studies. However, more extensive exploration of this link is required to identify the underlying modifiable risk factors. In the present study, one such factor, namely, emotion regulation difficulties, was explored to see its mediating effect in the relationship between neuroticism and HRBs—the first two constructs of the mentioned link. In this quantitative study, a total of 759 adolescents belonging to the Indian state of Punjab (Males= 402; *M*(age)=16.08) provided relevant information on a set of standardized questionnaires. Mediation analysis supported the major hypothesis of the present study. The results suggest that emotion regulation difficulty may be a significant mediator in the neuroticism-HRBs link. One's difficulty in regulating emotions might be an underlying mechanism through which high neuroticism increases the probability of indulging in HRBs, resulting in adverse health outcomes. The study implies that the assessment of emotion regulation difficulties should be included in interventional programs aimed at achieving adolescents' wellbeing, and early intervention may avoid progression toward adverse health outcomes in adulthood.

Over 1.5 million adolescents aged 10-24 years died in 2019, primarily due to preventable or treatable causes, including health-risk behaviors (World Health Organization, 2021). A health risk behavior is any behavior with a frequency or intensity that increases the risk of disease or injury with or without the awareness of the link between the behavior and the risk (Steptoe, 2007). These health-risk behaviors (HRBs) may be related to addictive behaviors (e.g. excessive alcohol consumption, smoking), externalizing behaviors (e.g. violence, self-harm) or unsafe sexual activities and sedentary lifestyle (e.g. physical inactivity and unhealthy dietary behaviors) (Underwood *et al.*, 2020). Some of these behaviors may continue into adulthood (Lee *et al.*, 2016), and some may even cause immediate death (Johns *et al.*, 2019). HRBs have become leading causes of mortality among adolescents, especially in low and middle-income countries

(Weiss & Ferrand, 2019). Mitigation of such adverse health outcomes requires researchers and policymakers to address biological, psychosocial, and environmental factors that underlie or maintain HRBs among adolescents. The success of the interventional programmes designed to promote health, such as '*The Global strategy for women's, children's and youths' wellbeing (2016–2030)*' (World Health Organization, 2015), depends on an adequate understanding of adolescence age, the causal mechanism of health-promoting behaviors and HRBs. The present study aimed to understand some aspects of HRBs among adolescents. In previous studies, various mechanisms through which adolescents acquire and maintain HRBs have been investigated. The present study explored the mediating effect of emotion regulation difficulties in the neuroticism-HRBs link. The knowledge generated may assist in designing the required plans to protect young people from engaging in HRBs.

The physiological, neurological, and psychosocial transformations during adolescence may drive the youth to engage in HRBs (Zimmermann *et al.*, 2019). However, adolescents do not adopt these HRBs in a vacuum, and various risk and protective factors determine their development and maintenance (Bailey *et al.*, 2019; Bozzini *et al.*, 2020). The Problem-Behavior Theory (Donovan *et al.*, 1993) suggests that the maladaptive behavioral pattern arises from an imbalance of three psychosocial factors, namely, personality (e.g. temperament, values, beliefs), environmental (e.g. family and peer expectations), and behavioral (coping behavioral patterns). These factors may drive some adolescents to acquire unhealthy and problematic behaviors like risky driving and drug abuse (Hirani *et al.*, 2018). Culture also plays an important role in regulating health-related behaviors (Hamzah *et al.*, 2019; Napier *et al.*, 2014); however, not many studies have empirically explored the role of culture on specific HRBs. Previous studies suggested that individuals' cultural context should be considered while targeting health behavior change (Higgins, 2014; Kaplan, 2014). The results imply that the nature of associations among different risk and protective factors for HRBs may vary in different cultures. Therefore, before devising any interventional programme for reducing HRBs, the cultural context of the targeted population should be addressed.

While considering the significance of HRBs for adverse health outcomes, researchers tried to understand the phenomenon and explored the potential risk factors for HRBs (Bailey *et al.*, 2019; Bozzini *et al.*, 2020). There are possibilities of multiple pathways leading to indulgence in HRBs, and one such potential pathway may involve neuroticism and emotion regulation difficulties. Researchers have been exploring the role of personality traits in influencing behavioral patterns; however, the role of personality traits in developing HRBs is still not very clear. The current study explored the association of a personality trait, namely neuroticism, with HRBs. Both direct and indirect effects (through emotion regulation difficulties) of neuroticism on different HRBs were explored.

Neuroticism has been linked with various physical and mental health issues (Malouff *et al.*, 2005, 2006, 2007); it has a substantial predictive utility for several mental health outcomes (Fanous *et al.*, 2007) and physical health problems (Smith & MacKenzie, 2006; Suls & Bunde, 2005). in a longitudinal study, Shipley *et al.* (2007; 21-year study with 5,424 adults) found that each *SD* unit increase in neuroticism at the baseline was associated with a 10% greater mortality from heart-related issues. However, previous studies concerning the relationship between neuroticism and health outcomes observed mixed or inconsistent findings. The discrepancies in the findings led to two types of explanations (Friedman, 2000) through which neuroticism might relate to health. First, neuroticism may lead to adverse health outcomes *via* increased indulgence in anxiety-provoked maladaptive and risky behaviors. Second, neuroticism may lead to good health due to vigilance provoked by anxiety. There is an urgent need for more research to clarify this discrepancy and expand the understanding of the neuroticism-health associations. For translating this understanding into a prevention model, the mediating and moderating factors that influence the neuroticism-health associations need to be explored. Among other mechanisms, previous studies supported the mediating role of HRBs in the relationship between neuroticism and adverse health outcomes (Smith & MacKenzie, 2006). The health behavior model of personality suggested that personality impacts health and mortality indirectly *via* specific behaviors (Turiano, 2012). Personality predisposes some individuals with specific traits to engage in one or the other form of HRBs (Murray & Booth, 2015). Many studies have observed a direct association between personality traits and various HRBs, such as smoking (Graham *et al.*, 2017), alcohol consumption (Turiano *et al.*, 2015), unprotected sex (Trobst *et al.*, 2000), and physical activity (Graham *et al.*, 2018). These behaviors further affect an individual's health and life expectancy.

Thus, the literature indicated that HRBs serve as mediators in the personality-health link; neuroticism leads to HRBs, and these behaviors further damage health and increase mortality risk (Turiano *et al.*, 2013, 2012; Weston & Jackson, 2016). The present study moved one step further to explore the association between neuroticism and HRBs, and emotion regulation difficulty was introduced as a mediator in the neuroticism-HRBs link. Thus, the present examined the role of emotion regulation difficulties as a mediator between neuroticism-HRBs link and wanted to explore whether neuroticism indirectly influences HRBs *via* emotion regulation difficulties. Mediation can be explored if all three variables under study are theoretically connected; neuroticism, emotion regulation difficulties, and HRBs should be related to each other. The relationship between neuroticism and HRBs have been supported in previous studies, some of which have already been presented in the previous paragraph. The relationship between neuroticism and emotion regulation has also been explored and established. However, most studies were conducted on the clinical sample, and only a few studies investigated the phenomenon on non-clinical samples (John & Gross, 2004; Purnamaningsih, 2017). The studies on non-clinical samples observed a strong association between the constructs. Higher levels of neuroticism were found to be significant predictors of emotion regulation difficulties (Kokkonen & Pulkkinen, 2001). Individuals high on neuroticism made fewer attempts to repair emotions to make them more adaptive and maintain positive affect. Similar findings have also been observed in other studies (e.g. Boland & Cappeliez, 1997; Vollrath *et al.*, 1995).

The direct association between emotion regulation and HRBs has also been established (e.g. Weiss *et al.*, 2015). Deficits in emotion regulation were found to be significantly related to HRBs (Gross, 2015). Emotion regulation has been conceptualized as a process of shaping which emotions one has and how one expresses these emotions to achieve the desired goal (De Berardis *et al.*, 2020; Gross, 2015; Thompson, 1994).

Emotion regulation comprises multiple skills, such as recognizing one's emotional state, identifying affect in others and using different adaptive strategies for moderating one's emotional reaction. When a person lacks the skills or fails to execute the skills appropriately, emotions become less effective. The process model of emotion regulation (Gross, 2015) has been widely used to explain the relationship between emotional dysregulation and HRBs (Webb *et al.*, 2012). The model suggested that individuals who cannot change their emotions to achieve a goal would feel distressed. The distress may further lead to various HRBs, such as drug abuse, alcohol abuse, sexual risk behaviors, bullying, aggressive behaviors, unhealthy dietary behaviors, addictive behaviors, unintentional injuries or violence-related behaviors, suicidal behaviors, and lack of medical adherence (Garofalo & Velotti, 2017; Lansing *et al.*, 2019; Ram *et al.*, 2018; Weiss *et al.*, 2015; Zafar *et al.*, 2021). In the past, different types of specific difficulties that individuals may experience while regulating ones' emotions have also been explored. In this regard, Gratz and Roemer (2004), based on a framework of experiential avoidance, devised a clinical model of difficulties in emotion regulation (Hayes *et al.*, 1996). The model stated that the difficulties that cause emotional disturbance are related to (a) understanding and acceptance of emotions, (b) the ability to refrain from impulsive behaviors (c) the utilization of adaptive ways to regulate the intensity and duration of emotional responses, and (d) ability to use emotional regulation strategies that are perceived to be effective for feeling better. The model suggested that the deficits in any of these processes may cause dysfunctional emotion regulation. Further, to deal with dysfunctional emotions, the individual may indulge in health-compromising behaviors, such as smoking, drugs, self-mutilating, and violence (Gratz & Roemer, 2004).

The previous studies showed that neuroticism could be a notable risk factor for indulgence in HRBs among adolescents. However, most of the studies primarily investigated the direct relationship between neuroticism and HRBs. To comprehensively understand the inter-construct mechanism, more studies are required to explore the role of specific/modifiable factors that mediate the relationship between neuroticism and HRBs (Lozano-Madrid *et al.*, 2020). This understanding can be a good value addition for future interventions to prevent adolescents' indulgence in HRBs. Among other factors, emotion regulation difficulties may be studied as a potential mediator because: 1) neuroticism has been linked to emotional dysregulation (Kokkonen & Pulkkinen, 2001), and 2) emotion dysregulation is considered a potentially transdiagnostic process of many forms of psychopathology as well as health-related issues and has been linked to HRBs (Fu *et al.*, 2020; Zafar *et al.*, 2021). In other words, as emotion regulation has been associated with both the antecedent (neuroticism) and consequent condition (HRBs), it may have some mediational role in the neuroticism-HRBs link. Identification of such roles in the neuroticism-HRBs link may indicate an alternative approach to target HRBs.

The Present Study

As the literature suggests, adolescence is generally associated with a higher risk-taking tendency (Arnett & Balle-Jensen, 1993; Jessor, 1991; Smith *et al.*, 2014; van den Bos & Hertwig, 2017). However, the tendency to indulge in HRBs vary among adolescents, and not all adolescents indulge in HRBs. Various risk and protective factors associated with personality and environment can make an individual more or less vulnerable to HRBs than another individual (Jessor, 1991). The present study was an effort to explore the nature of relationships among potentially significant factors associated with HRBs, which may explain the individual differences in the vulnerabilities for HRBs. More specifically, the present study intended to provide empirical information about the nature of the relationships between neuroticism, emotion regulation difficulties and HRBs. It was mainly carried out to explore the mediating role of emotion regulation difficulties in the neuroticism-HRBs relationship. In the study, the summated effect of six types of difficulties in emotion regulation, namely, lack of emotional awareness, lack of emotional clarity, difficulties engaging in goal-directed behavior, impulse control difficulties, limited access to effective emotion-regulation strategies, and non-acceptance of emotional responses, was explored with regard to four types of HRBs, namely, risky driving, violence, self-harm, unhealthy dietary behavior & physical inactivity. Based on the literature review, it was hypothesized that neuroticism would be positively associated with all HRBs(H1), emotion regulation difficulties would be positively associated with HRBs(H2), and emotion regulation difficulties would mediate the association between neuroticism and HRBs(H3). Further, it was also expected that neuroticism and emotion regulation difficulties would be strongly related to self-harm and violence more than the other two HRBs, namely, risky driving and unhealthy dietary behavior & physical inactivity.

Method

Sample

This study's sample, procured using a multi-stage stratified sampling, consisted of 759 (Males= 402) participants in the age group of 15-18 years (Mean age = 16.08, SD= 0.97). The study protocol was approved by the Institute Ethics Committee (Human). The participants were selected from different schools of five districts of the Indian state of Punjab. The participants were enrolled in 9-12th grades and belonged to both rural and urban areas of Punjab. Four schools from each district and 40 students from each school were selected using the fishbowl technique. In the present COVID-19 crisis, the relevant information was obtained using online forms. The study's purpose and procedure were clarified to education offices, school authorities, study participants, and parents. Following these, the participants were asked to confirm their willingness to participate in the present study. As the study participants were minors, informed consent was obtained from parents or guardians also. Out of 800 students selected for the study, only 759 participants and their parents gave consent. The distribution of participants within the sample in terms of sex, class, and locality has been presented in Table 1.

Measures

In the current study, the relevant questions from the Youth Risk Behavior Survey Questionnaire (YRBSS; Centre for Disease Control & Prevention, 2019) were taken

Table 1. Demographic Characteristics of the Total Sample and Descriptive Statistics.

Demographic characteristics	N	%age	Min.	Max.	Mean	SD	Skewness	Kurtosis
Age (Years)	759		15	18	16.08	0.97	0.39	−0.93
Gender								
Male	402	53.0						
Female	357	47.0						
Education								
9th	144	19.0						
10th	187	24.6						
11th	192	25.3						
12th	236	31.1						
Locality								
Rural	371	48.9						
Urban	388	51.1						
Scores on the Neuroticism scale	759		12	60	35.21	5.98	−0.02	1.00
Scores on the Emotion regulation difficulties scale	759		36	162	93.94	23.64	0.17	−0.41
Scores on the Risky-Driving subscale	759		0	4	0.94	0.74	1.02	2.30
Scores on the Violence subscale	759		0	6	0.79	1.24	2.04	4.42
Scores on the Self-Harm subscale	759		0	5	0.51	0.79	2.35	6.33
Scores on the Unhealthy Dietary and Physical Inactivity subscale	759		0	13	6.92	2.40	−0.04	−0.38

and used to assess participants' engagement in selected HRBs. Besides, the NEO-FFI (Costa & McCrae, 1992) and the Difficulties in Emotion Regulation Questionnaire (Gratz & Roemer, 2004) were used in their original form.

Youth Risk Behavior Survey Questionnaire

The Youth Risk Behavior Survey (Centre for Disease Control & Prevention, 2019) was used to assess the presence and severity of HRBs among adolescents. This questionnaire is a part of the Youth Risk Behavior Surveillance System, an annual assessment initiated by the Center for Disease Control and Prevention. The Youth Risk Behavior Surveillance System (YRBSS) monitors a few categories of significant health-related behaviors among adolescents and young adults, for instance, risky driving, violence, self-harm, unhealthy dietary behaviors & physical inactivity. The YRBSS standard questionnaire contains 89 questions, but in the present study, only 31 items were used to assess the four types of HRBs. Higher scores on each type indicate a higher indulgence in the risk behaviors. In a recent study on a large sample (Lima *et al.*, 2020), the psychometric properties of the scale were found satisfactory; Cronbach's alpha was found to be 0.77 for the overall scale, and most of the domains (82%) showed intraclass correlation coefficient to be more than 0.75. In the present study, the overall Cronbach alpha was 0.73 and domain-wise, it varied from 0.69 to 0.78. Some representative items of the questionnaire are: "During the past 30 days, how many times did you drive/ride a car/scooter or another vehicle faster than the prescribed speed limit"; "During the past 12 months, how many times were you in a physical fight in the school?"; "During the past 12 months, did you intentionally harm yourself physically?"; "During the past seven days, on how many days did you eat meals on time?"; "During the past seven days, on how many days were you physically active for a total of at least 60 min per day?"

The NEO Five-Factor Inventory (NEO-FFI)

The NEO- FFI (Costa & McCrae, 1992) was used to measure adolescents' personality characteristics. It is a 60-item inventory that measures five domains of personality, namely, Neuroticism, Extraversion, Openness, Agreeableness, and Conscientiousness. Each subscale includes 12 self-descriptive statements on a 5-point Likert-type scale ranging from 'strongly disagree' to 'strongly agree'. Scores for each domain are calculated by summing the 12 responses after adjusting the scoring for reversed items. The reliability and validity of the inventory have been established in previous studies conducted across the cultures; Cronbach-alpha in most of the studies ranged from 0.68 to 0.85 (Sherry *et al.*, 2007). In the present study, only the neuroticism subscale of the inventory was used. A representative item of the neuroticism subscale is: "Too often, when things go wrong, I get discouraged and feel like giving up". For the present sample, the Cronbach alpha for the neuroticism subscale was 0.78.

Difficulties in Emotion Regulation Questionnaire

Difficulties in Emotion Regulation Questionnaire (Gratz & Roemer, 2004), a 36-item self-report measure, assess individuals' characteristic levels of overall emotion regulation difficulties and six specific difficulties, namely, non-acceptance of emotional responses, difficulties engaging in goal-directed behaviors when distressed, difficulties controlling impulsive behaviors when distressed, lack of emotional awareness, limited access to emotion regulation strategies perceived as effective and lack of emotional clarity. Respondents are required to indicate *how often* the items apply to themselves, with options ranging from 'almost never' to 'almost always'. Some representative items are: "When I am upset, I know that I can find a way to eventually feel better" (Reversed scored) and "When I am upset, I have difficulty getting work done." The total score ranges from 36-180, and the higher scores indicate more difficulties in emotion regulation. In terms of reliability, the overall DERS score and the subscale scores have been found to have high internal consistency. For instance, the values of the coefficient for lack of awareness, lack of clarity, lack of goal-directed behavior, difficulty in controlling impulsive behavior, non-acceptance, and lack of emotional strategies were found to be 0.82, 0.82, 0.86, 0.88, 0.92, 0.95, respectively (Hallion *et al.*, 2018). In the present study, a summated score of all 36 items was used to measure emotion regulation difficulties, and the Cronbach alpha came out to be 0.91.

Procedure

First of all, the researcher submitted the research proposal to the Institute Ethics Committee (Human) for ethics clearance, and the committee approved the same through letter no. IEC/11/2019. After preparing the required questionnaire set, a statistical power analysis was performed for sample size estimation. Based on the effect sizes mentioned in previous studies, a small effect size of 0.15 (Cohen, 1988) was expected. With an alpha = .01 and power = 0.80, a sample of a minimum of 698 participants was considered sufficient for small effect size (Cohen, 1992). Thus, the sample size of the present study ($N = 759$) was adequate for the purpose. In the present study, multi-stage stratified sampling was used to select participants. There are twenty-three districts in Punjab spread in three geological strata: Majha, Malwa, and Doaba. Malwa, the largest, covers 14 districts. The other two regions have four districts in each. Out of these districts, five districts in total, namely, Bathinda, Patiala, Ropar (Malwa), Jalandhar (Doaba) and Gurdaspur (Majha), were selected randomly. The present study was carried out in three phases.

In the first phase, the researcher contacted local district education officers (DEOs) of the mentioned districts. The DEOs provided relevant lists of various schools, including rural and urban schools. From a complete list of 323 schools, initially, 100 schools (20 schools from each selected district) were randomly selected. The researcher then contacted the selected schools ' Principals, coordinators and school counselors and provided them with detailed information about the project, either telephonically or through emails. Based on the responses, four schools from each district were finally shortlisted for data collection. In the second phase, the researcher conducted orientation webinars or the teachers, coordinators and counselors, wherein the nature of the present study was explained. The school authorities provided the contact details of the parents. Parents were then contacted either telephonically or through emails and were informed about the study. Later, an online consent form was sent containing information about all the potential risks and benefits of participating in the study. Parents were first asked to read the information given and then indicate their decision to permit or not to permit their children to participate. Those who gave their consent were requested to provide the details of their children. Upon submission of the parental consent form, the selected questionnaires were sent to their children, the main participants of the study. All questionnaires were used in their original English language. In order to rule out any language-related bias, all the participants were initially asked about their English language proficiency, especially in reading and comprehension. Most of the participants (students) had been receiving their class instructions in the English language for at least five years. Participants did not report any difficulty in understanding the questions. A total of 800 participants were contacted; a few parents did not provide due consent. After removing partially filled questionnaires, a total of 759 observations could be used for the statistical analysis. In the final phase, once the targeted responses were received from a particular school, webinars-cum-workshops were conducted for the participants by trained psychologists as partial compensation for their participation.

Statistical Analysis

Before conducting mediation analyses, the researcher verified the prerequisite conditions for the same; relationships between (1) neuroticism and HRBs, (2) neuroticism and emotion regulation difficulties, and (3) emotion regulation difficulties and HRBs were evaluated. Then, in order to test the stated hypotheses, the authors conducted the mediation analyses to obtain the indirect effects of neuroticism on all HRBs (mediation effects; through path analysis using IBM SPSS AMOS 25.0). Mediation occurs when a predictor (neuroticism) affects a dependent variable (HRBs) indirectly through at least one intervening variable (the mediator; Preacher & Hayes, 2008). Additionally, the hierarchical regression analysis was also applied to explore the relative importance of both the constructs in predicting HRBs and confirm the mediation.

Results

The findings of the present study are summarized in four tables and one figure. Table 1 shows the demographic characteristics of the sample and descriptive statistics. A total of 402 (53%) males and 357 (47%) females participated in this study. The mean age of all the participants was 16.08 ± 0.97 (15-18) years (Table 1). Table 2 presents the correlation coefficients (controlled for age and gender) among the studied variables. Significant positive correlations were observed among scores on neuroticism, emotion regulation difficulties and HRBs. Scores on neuroticism subscale (the predictor) were significantly correlated with scores on risky-driving subscale, r (759) =0.11, p<.01, violence, r (759) =0.18, p<.01, self-harm, r (759) =0.25, p<.01, and unhealthy dietary and physical activities, r (759) =0.08, p=.04 (Table 2); the findings were consistent with previous studies (e.g. Drossman *et al.*, 2000; Fanous *et al.*, 2007). Neuroticism came out to be associated with the emotion regulation difficulties also (the mediator), r (759) =0.38, p<.01 (Table 2), as found in the literature (Kokkonen & Pulkkinen, 2001; Purnamaningsih, 2017). Similarly, emotion regulation difficulties (the mediator) correlated significantly with risky driving, r (759) =0.15, p<.01, violence, r (759) =0.26, p<.01, self-harm, r (759) =0.37, p<.01, and unhealthy dietary and physical activities, r (759) =0.11, p=.004 (Table 2), as observed in previous studies (e.g. Garofalo & Velotti, 2017; Weiss *et al.*, 2015). Thus, the first two hypotheses were supported by the present data. Neuroticism, as well as emotion regulation difficulties, were significantly associated with HRBs. As expected, neuroticism and emotion regulation difficulties were related more strongly to self-harm and violence than the other two HRBs, namely, risky driving and unhealthy dietary behavior & physical inactivity.

Testing of the third hypothesis (H3) required mediation analysis. For this purpose, the researcher used a mediation testing approach suggested by Preacher and Hayes (2004). Table 3 summarizes the findings of the mediation analysis and presents the standardized total, direct (of neuroticism controlling emotion regulation difficulties) and indirect effects of neuroticism (through emotion regulation difficulties) on four types of HRBs. The *standardized direct effects* of neuroticism (β values) on self-harm, risky driving, violence and unhealthy dietary and physical activities came out to be 0.13, 0.05, 0.09 and 0.04, respectively (Table 3). Similarly, the *standardized indirect effects* (β values; mediated through emotion regulation difficulties) of neuroticism on self-harm, risky driving, violence and unhealthy dietary and physical activities came out to be 0.13, 0.05, 0.08 and 0.05, respectively (Table 3). That means, due to neuroticism's indirect (mediated) effect on the given HRBs, when neuroticism increased by one standard deviation, engagement in the studies HRBs decreased by 0.13, 0.05, 0.08 and 0.05 standard deviations, respectively. This effect was in addition to any direct (unmediated) effect that neuroticism might have on all these HRBs. As shown, the indirect effects of neuroticism for HRBs came out to be statistically significant.

The standardized indirect (mediated) effects of neuroticism on studied HRBs were significantly different from zero at the 0.01 level (two-tailed; p=.003, p= .006, p=.003

Table 2. Correlation Coefficients Among Scores on Neuroticism, Emotion Regulation Difficulties and Four Types of Health-Risk Behaviors.

Variables	1	2	3	4	5	6
1 Neuroticism	1.00					
2 Emotion Regulation Difficulties	0.39**	1.00				
3 Risky-Driving	0.10**	0.14**	1.00			
4 Violence	0.17**	0.24**	0.35**	1.00		
5 Self-Harm	0.26**	0.39**	0.13**	0.31**	1.00	
6 Unhealthy Dietary and Physical Activities	0.09*	0.13**	0.12**	0.08*	0.12**	1.00

Note. $N=759$.
*$p<0.05$.
**$p<0.01$.

Table 3. Standardized Total, Direct (of Neuroticism Controlling Emotion Regulation Difficulties) and Indirect Effects for Four Types of Health-Risk Behaviors.

Variables	Total effect Neuroticism & Emotion regulation difficulties		Direct effect (Neuroticism)		Indirect effect	
	Estimates	p-value*	Estimates	p-value	Estimates	p-value
Self-Harm	0.26	0.003	0.13	0.005	0.13	0.003
Risky-Driving	0.10	0.014	0.05	0.221	0.05	0.006
Violence	0.17	0.005	0.09	0.007	0.08	0.003
Unhealthy Dietary and Physical Activities	0.09	0.014	0.04	0.221	0.05	0.004

Note. $N=759$.

and p=.004, respectively; Table 3). Though the indirect effects were significant for all HRBs, the findings indicated full mediation only for two types of HRBs, (risky driving and unhealthy dietary & physical activities). For these two types of HRBs, when total effects were partitioned, the direct effect could not reach the significance level (direct effects; p=.221 and p= .221, respectively; Table 3), but indirect effects were significant (indirect effects; p=.006 and p=.004, respectively; Table 3). For the remaining two types of HRBs, namely, violence and self-harm, mediation of emotion regulation difficulties for the neuroticism-HRBs link came out to be partial because the direct effects of neuroticism were significant (direct effects; p=.007 and p= .005, respectively; Table 3) even after partitioning the total effects. Thus, the findings showed that the emotion regulation difficulties fully mediate risky driving and unhealthy dietary and physical activities; however, the other two HRBs, namely, violence and self-harm, were partially mediated by emotion regulation difficulties. Figure 1 depicts the findings of the mediation analysis. The figure shows three types of paths (a, b & c) wherein path *a* represents standardized regression coefficient for the predictor in relation to the mediator. Path *b1, b2, b3* and *b4* represent standardized regression coefficients for the mediator predicting the given criterion variables. Path *c1, c2, c3* and *c4* are the direct effects representing standardized regression coefficients for the predictor in relation to criterion variables while controlling for the effect of the mediator. Values in the parentheses are the total effects of predictor and mediator on the criterion variables.

Additionally, the researcher also applied hierarchical regression analysis to explore the relative importance of both constructs in predicting HRBs and confirm the mediation; Table 4 summarizes the findings of the analysis. As shown, for each HRB, two

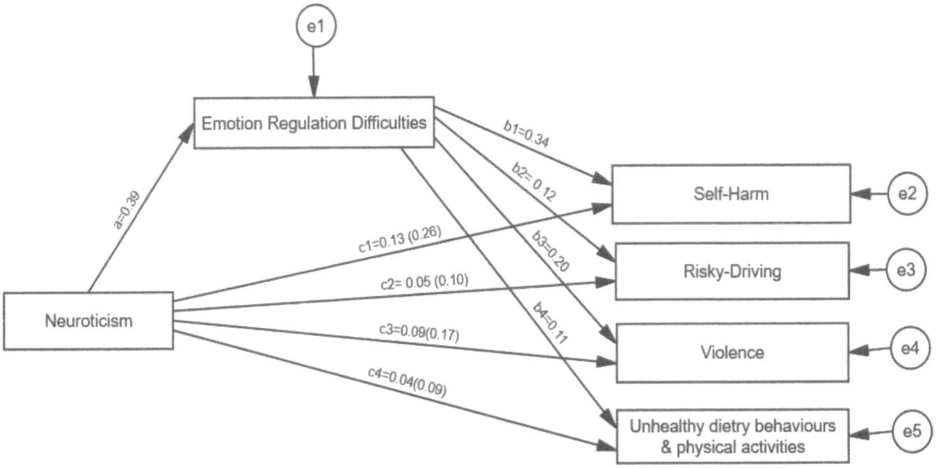

Figure 1. Neuroticism predicting health-risk behaviors with emotion regulation difficulties as a mediator. *Note.* Path a = standardized regression coefficient for the predictor in relation to the mediator; path b1-b4 = Standardized regression coefficient for the mediator predicting the criterion variables; path c1-c4 = standardized regression coefficient for the predictor in relation to criterion variables with the mediator in the model (direct effect); total effects are in parentheses.

separate regression analyses were conducted; in the first one, initially, neuroticism scores were introduced, followed by emotion regulation difficulties. In the second one, this order was reversed. The findings showed that the scores on emotion regulation difficulties were more strongly associated (depicted by the higher values of beta coefficients in Model 1) with all the criterion variables than the neuroticism scores. The second significant finding was that the beta values of neuroticism reduced after adding emotion regulation difficulties in the second model, indicating and confirming the mediating effect of emotion regulation difficulties in the neuroticism-HRBs link. The effect was not observed when neuroticism was added in the second model; not much change in emotion regulation difficulties betas was observed upon adding neuroticism in the equation. For instance, after adding scores on emotion regulation difficulties in the model, the beta value of neuroticism for risky driving reduced from $\beta = 0.096$, $t(757) = 2.65$, $p < 0.001$ to $\beta = 0.051$, $t(756) = 1.31$, $p = 0.190$ (Table 4), and it made the β (neuroticism) statistically non-significant. However, when the scores on neuroticism were added in the model, the beta value of emotion regulation difficulties for risky driving reduced marginally from $\beta = 0.136$, $t(757) = 3.77$, $p < 0.001$ to $\beta = 0.116$, $t(756) = 2.97$, $p = 0.003$ (Table 4) and the β(emotion regulation difficulties) remained statistically significant. Similar directions were observed for other HRBs also.

Discussion

Through the present study, the researcher intended to explore the nature of the relationship among two important factors associated with HRBs. Specifically, the current study mainly explored the mediating role of emotion regulation difficulties in the

Table 4. Hierarchical Regression for Health Risk Behaviors with Neuroticism and Emotion Regulation Difficulties as Predictors.

Criterion Variables	Order of Predictors	Model 1			Model 2		
		Unstandardized Coefficients		Standardized Coefficients	Unstandardized Coefficients		Standardized Coefficients
		B	SE(B)	β(p-value)	B	SE(B)	β(p-value)
Risky Driving	Neuroticism	0.010	0.005	0.096 **(0.008)**	0.006	0.005	0.051 **(0.190)**
	ERD		----		0.004	0.001	0.116
	ERD	0.004	0.001	0.136 **(0.000)**	0.004	0.001	0.116 **(0.003)**
	Neuroticism		----		0.006	0.005	0.051
Violence	Neuroticism	0.035	0.007	0.169 **(0.000)**	0.019	0.008	0.090 **(0.020)**
	ERD		----		0.110	0.002	0.205
	ERD	0.013	0.002	0.240 **(0.000)**	0.110	0.002	0.205 **(0.000)**
	Neuroticism		----		0.019	0.008	0.090
Self-Harm	Neuroticism	0.039	0.005	0.259 **(0.000)**	0.019	0.005	0.127 **(0.000)**
	ERD		----		0.013	0.001	0.341
	ERD	0.015	0.001	0.390 **(0.000)**	0.013	0.001	0.341**(0.000)**
	Neuroticism		----		0.019	0.005	0.127
Unhealthy Dietary and Physical Activities	Neuroticism	0.035	0.015	0.087 **(0.017)**	0.018	0.016	0.044 **(0.263)**
	ERD		----		0.011	0.004	0.112
	ERD	0.013	0.004	0.129 **(0.000)**	0.011	0.004	0.112 **(0.004)**
	Neuroticism		----		0.018	0.016	0.044

Note. $N = 759$.
ERD-Emotion Regulation Difficulties.

neuroticism-HRBs link among adolescents. The researcher predicted that neuroticism, emotion regulation difficulties, and HRBs would correlate positively, and emotion regulation difficulties would mediate the relationship between neuroticism and HRBs. As hypothesized, emotion regulation difficulties came out to be a significant mediator. However, it partially mediated the said relationship for two specific HRBs, namely, violence and self-harm. The present study's findings indicate that one's difficulty in regulating emotions may be an underlying mechanism through which high neuroticism increases the probability of indulging in various forms of HRBs that may subsequently lead to severe adverse health outcomes.

Adolescence, characterized as a period of storm and stress, has been associated with a higher risk-taking tendency in the youth. Certain specific experiences that occur mainly during adolescence, such as the need for excitement, peer pressure, egocentrism and perceived invulnerability, may predispose adolescence to indulge in risk-taking behaviors (Arnett & Balle-Jensen, 1993; Jessor, 1991; Smith *et al.*, 2014; van den Bos & Hertwig, 2017). However, the tendency to indulge in HRBs vary among adolescents, and not all adolescents indulge in HRBs. Various risk and protective factors associated with personality and environment make an individual more or less vulnerable to HRBs than another individual (Jessor, 1991). Identification of such factors that impact engagement in HRBs may have important implications. Moreover, exploring the mediation effects of the variables is crucial in providing alternate explanations for the outcomes as it can clarify why or how a direct association occurs between a predictor and the criterion variable. Identification and intervention at this early age may prevent adolescents from getting into severe risky behaviors.

The present study's findings extend support to the previous studies showing a significant direct relationship between neuroticism and HRBs (Drossman *et al.*, 2000; Fanous *et al.*, 2007; Smith & MacKenzie, 2006; Suls & Bunde, 2005). However, when the mediator variable (emotion regulation difficulties) was included in the equation, the direct effect of neuroticism became non-significant for risky driving and unhealthy dietary and physical activities. For the other two HRBs, both direct and indirect effects came out to be significant.

The significant mediation of emotion regulation difficulties, to some extent, support the assumption that neuroticism may not be fully and directly associated with HRBs (Friedman, 2000), but it relates to HRBs *via* emotion regulation difficulties. Relevant empirical and theoretical research work can help explain the mediational dynamics observed for neuroticism and HRBs relationship. Among various explanations provided by previous research works, one perspective maintained that individuals high in neuroticism in general experience more negative affect (anxiety, depression) and stress as compared to individuals low in neuroticism (Mroczek & Almeida, 2004; Suls *et al.*, 1998; Watson & Clark, 1994). When the negative emotions and stress are not regulated effectively (due to deficit in emotion regulation skills), individuals may indulge in poor health behaviors such as self-harm, violence, smoking, alcohol abuse to alleviate heightened negative emotions (Friedman, 2000; Smith, 2006). According to John and Gross (2004), individuals low in neuroticism experience fewer and less strong negative emotions and, as a result, are not required to deal with consequences of negative affectivity. This state may make it easier for individuals low in neuroticism to use adaptive and effective regulation strategies early in the process of emotion generation than it is for individuals high in neuroticism (John & Gross, 2004). So, the susceptibility of individuals high in neuroticism to experience more negative affect may further deteriorate their emotion regulation capabilities. It may lead to more indulgence in the HRBs to alleviate their chronically high levels of perceived stress and negative affect (Eysenck, 1973, 1991). This self-medication, though it provides short-term psychological relief, has a physical health cost. Thus, it is assumed that neuroticism makes an individual susceptible to experiencing more negative emotions, but it may be the inability to regulate one's negative emotions that drive them to indulge in HRBs. In a longitudinal study, Kokkonen and Pulkkinen (2001) found a significant association between neuroticism and emotion regulation deficits; higher levels of neuroticism contributed to higher levels of emotion regulation deficits. Individuals high in neuroticism made fewer attempts to repair emotions toward a positive direction and were more inclined to engage in HRBs as a means of attenuating negative affective states (Kokkonen & Pulkkinen, 2001).

Gray's Behavioral Inhibition System (BIS; Gray, 1981, 1988, 1994) explained why people high in neuroticism experience greater negative affect and stress and consequently engage more in HRBs. According to this model, it is the threat sensitivity that underlies the activation of negative emotion and behavioral withdrawal. Some individuals have more sensitive BIS than others, making them more responsive to real or perceived threats—these persons are generally high in neuroticism (Gray, 1994). Therefore, these hypersensitive individuals are more likely to get into HRBs to alleviate the unpleasantness that arises from BIS activation. Another theory of self-regulation

(Carver & Scheier, 1990; 1998) mentioned the existence of monitoring systems that provide feedback to the individual. In a perceived negative scenario, the monitoring systems will activate negative emotions, further leading to poor health behaviors. Such behaviors alleviate the negative feelings and reinforce such indulgence in the future (Cooper *et al.*, 2000).

Mediation of emotion regulation difficulties between neuroticism and HRBs can be explained with another observation that persons high in neuroticism use more emotion-focused and less problem-focused strategies (Watson & Hubbard, 1996) and are more likely to use inefficient escape-avoidance strategies to cope with stress (Bolger, 1990). Thus, it appears that persons high in neuroticism have an increased likelihood of experiencing negative emotions which they cannot manage effectively, leading to more negative affect and subsequent indulgence in risky behaviors as an alternative means of attenuating negative affect (Cicchetti *et al.*, 1995; Thompson, 1994). The present study indicates the possibility of poor emotion regulation leading to HRBs rather than the emotional susceptibility of individuals high in neuroticism. The direct effect of neuroticism has been challenged previously also where the interaction of neuroticism with other variables was found to be more significant than the main effect of neuroticism. For instance, predictive effects of neuroticism were found to be moderated by conscientiousness (Weston *et al.*, 2019), socioeconomic status and gender (Hagger-Johnson *et al.*, 2012). Many studies observed that high conscientiousness and high neuroticism were associated with lower indulgence in HRBs (Weston & Jackson, 2015, Turiano *et al.*, 2012). In contrast, high neuroticism and low conscientiousness were associated with greater indulgence in HRBs (Vollrath & Torgersen, 2002). Thus, these observations may be taken for further consideration that the direct effect of neuroticism may be less significant than its indirect effects.

Conclusion, Implications and Recommendations

The present study's findings highlight the significance of emotion regulation difficulties for different forms of HRBs among adolescents of Punjab. The study expands the literature about the mediational dynamics of neuroticism-HRBs link, which may further help future researchers to develop prevention and intervention programs targeting the emotional regulation skills of individuals indulging in HRBs. In other words, the findings imply that some forms of emotion regulation interventions can reduce adolescents' tendency to indulge in these HRBs. Supporting this implication, Houck *et al.* (2016) assessed the efficacy of emotion regulation intervention in reducing indulgence in violence and sexual risk behavior and observed a significant effect of the intervention. However, more studies are required to explore emotion regulation difficulties elaborately and assess the efficacy of training programmes to manage the same for a wider range of HRBs. Interventions targeting emotion dysregulation may help adolescents deal with dysfunctional emotions, and subsequently, a reduction in HRB can be expected. Training programmes to be tested may include emotion awareness modules that sensitize adolescents about the role of emotion regulation styles in promoting mental and physical health. Besides, skill training for a few compatible and adaptive emotion regulation strategies, with the ultimate goal of increasing emotional clarity, healthy expression and acceptance of emotions, should be included. The assessment of emotion regulation difficulties should also be included in all the preventive and interventional programs aimed to achieve adolescents' physical and psychological well-being. Early intervention should be provided to avoid progression toward HRBs in adulthood.

Limitations

The findings of this study should be generalized cautiously due to some inherent limitations. As the measures utilized in this study are self-report measures, the possibilities of socially desirable responses cannot be ruled out. However, the self-report technique should be more helpful as individuals can better state their emotional experiences and behavioral reactions than external observers (Raine *et al.*, 2006). Besides, low mean scores of some HRBs and slight deviance from normality might have affected the correlation coefficients. Language related concerns may also be a limitation of the study. Though the English proficiency was ensured and the questions were not hard to understand, some participants might still have difficulty understanding any non-native language. The multi-level analysis, including more predictors such as other personality factors and environmental factors including home environment and parenting styles, might have provided a better understanding of studied HRBs.

Disclosure Statement

No potential conflict of interest was reported by the author.

Ethical Statement

The research reported in the manuscript was conducted in accordance with general ethical guidelines in psychology. Ethics clearance was provided by the Institute Ethics Committee (Human) through letter no. IEC/11/2019.

Funding

The study was funded by the Indian Council of Medical Research, New Delhi (India) through Grant no. Adhoc/136/2019/HSR.

ORCID

Parwinder Singh http://orcid.org/0000-0002-6026-5815

Data Availability Statement

The data that support the findings of this study are available from the corresponding author upon reasonable request.

References

Arnett, J., & Balle-Jensen, L. (1993). Cultural Bases of Risk Behavior: Danish Adolescents. *Child Development, 64*(6), 1842–1855. https://doi.org/10.1111/j.1467-8624.1993.tb04217.x

Bailey, J. M., Regan, T. W., Bartlem, K. M., Wiggers, J. H., Wye, P. M., & Bowman, J. A. (2019). A survey of the prevalence of modifiable health risk behaviours among carers of people with a mental illness. *BMC Public Health, 19*(1), 1–10. https://doi.org/10.1186/s12889-019-7577-4

Boland, A., & Cappeliez, P. (1997). Optimism and neuroticism as predictors of coping and adaptation in older women. *Personality and Individual Differences, 22*(6), 909–919. https://doi.org/10.1016/S0191-8869(96)00251-6

Bolger, N. (1990). Coping as a personality process: A prospective study. *Journal of Personality and Social Psychology, 59*(3), 525–537. https://doi.org/10.1037/0022-3514.59.3.525

Bozzini, A. B., Bauer, A., Maruyama, J., Simões, R., & Matijasevich, A. (2020). Factors associated with risk behaviors in adolescence: A systematic review. *Brazilian Journal of Psychiatry, 43*(2), 210–221. https://doi.org/10.1590/1516-4446-2019-0835

Carver, C. S., & Scheier, M. F. (1990). Origins and functions of positive and negative affect: A control-process view. *Psychological Review, 97*(1), 19–35. https://doi.org/10.1037/0033-295X.97.1.19

Carver, C. S., & Scheier, M. F. (1998). *On the self-regulation of behavior* (1st ed.). Cambridge University Press.

Centre for Disease Control and Prevention. (2019). *Youth Risk Behavior Survey: Data summary & trends report 2007–2017.* https://www.cdc.gov/healthyyouth/data/yrbs/pdf/trendsreport.pdf.

Cicchetti, D., Ackerman, B. P., & Izard, C. E. (1995). Emotions and emotion regulation in developmental psychopathology. *Development and Psychopathology, 7*(1), 1–10. https://doi.org/10.1017/S0954579400006301

Cohen, J. (1988). *Statistical power analysis for the behavioral sciences.* L. Erlbaum Associates.

Cohen, J. (1992). Statistical Power Analysis. *Current Directions in Psychological Science, 1*(3), 98–101. https://doi.org/10.1111/1467-8721.ep10768783

Cooper, M. L., Agocha, V. B., & Sheldon, M. S. (2000). A motivational perspective on risky behaviors: The role of personality and affect regulatory processes. *Journal of Personality, 68*(6), 1059–1088. https://doi.org/10.1111/1467-6494.00126

Costa, P. T., & McCrae, R. R. (1992). *NEO PI-R: Professional manual. Revised NEO personality inventory NEO PR-R and NEO five-factor inventory NEO-RRI.* Psychological Assessment Resources.

De Berardis, D., Fornaro, M., Orsolini, L., Ventriglio, A., Vellante, F., & Di Giannantonio, M. (2020). Emotional dysregulation in adolescents: Implications for the development of severe psychiatric disorders, substance abuse, and suicidal ideation and behaviors. *Brain Sciences, 10*(9), 591. https://doi.org/10.3390/brainsci10090591

Donovan, J. E., Jessor, R., & Costa, F. M. (1993). Structure of health-enhancing behavior in adolescence: A latent-variable approach. *Journal of Health and Social Behavior, 34*(4), 346–362. https://doi.org/10.2307/2137372

Drossman, D. A., Leserman, J., Li, Z., Keefe, F., Hu, Y. J. B., & Toomey, T. C. (2000). Effects of coping on health outcome among women with gastrointestinal disorders. *Psychosomatic Medicine, 62*(3), 309–317. https://doi.org/10.1097/00006842-200005000-00004

Eysenck, H. (1973). Personality and the maintenance of the smoking habit. In W. L. Dunn (Ed.), *Smoking behavior: motives and incentives* (pp. 113–146). Winston.

Eysenck, H. J. (1991). *Smoking, personality, and stress: Psychosocial factors in the prevention of cancer and coronary heart disease*. Springer.

Fanous, A. H., Neale, M. C., Aggen, S. H., & Kendler, K. S. (2007). A longitudinal study of personality and major depression in a population-based sample of male twins. *Psychological Medicine, 37*(8), 1163–1172. https://doi.org/10.1017/S0033291707000244

Friedman, H. S. (2000). Long-term relations of personality and health: dynamisms, mechanisms, tropisms . *Journal of Personality, 68*(6), 1089–1107. https://doi.org/10.1111/1467-6494.00127

Fu, L., Wang, P., Zhao, M., Xie, X., Chen, Y., Nie, J., & Lei, L. (2020). Can emotion regulation difficulty lead to adolescent problematic smartphone use? A moderated mediation model of depression and perceived social support. *Children and Youth Services Review, 108*, 104660. https://doi.org/10.1016/j.childyouth.2019.104660

Garofalo, C., & Velotti, P. (2017). Negative emotionality and aggression in violent offenders: The moderating role of emotion dysregulation. *Journal of Criminal Justice, 51*, 9–16. https://doi.org/10.1016/j.jcrimjus.2017.05.015

Graham, E. K., Bastarache, E. D., Milad, E., Turiano, N. A., Cotter, K. A., & Mroczek, D. K. (2018). Physical activity mediates the association between personality and biomarkers of inflammation. *SAGE Open Medicine, 6*, 2050312118774990. https://doi.org/10.1177/2050312118774990

Graham, E. K., Rutsohn, J. P., Turiano, N. A., Bendayan, R., Batterham, P. J., Gerstorf, D., Katz, M. J., Reynolds, C. A., Sharp, E. S., Yoneda, T. B., Bastarache, E. D., Elleman, L. G., Zelinski, E. M., Johansson, B., Kuh, D., Barnes, L. L., Bennett, D. A., Deeg, D. J. H., Lipton, R. B., … Mroczek, D. K. (2017). Personality predicts mortality risk: An integrative data analysis of 15 international longitudinal studies. *Journal of Research in Personality, 70*, 174–186. https://doi.org/10.1016/j.jrp.2017.07.005

Gratz, K. L., & Roemer, L. (2004). Multidimensional assessment of emotion regulation and dysregulation: Development, factor structure, and initial validation of the difficulties in emotion regulation scale. *Journal of Psychopathology and Behavioral Assessment, 26*(1), 41–54. https://doi.org/10.1007/s10862-008-9102-4

Gray, J. A. (1981). A critique of Eysenck's theory of personality. In H. J. Eysenck (Ed.), *A model for personality* (pp. 246–276). Springer.

Gray, J. A. (1988). *The psychology of fear and stress (problems in the behavioural sciences, Series Number 5)* (2nd ed.). Cambridge University Press.

Gray, J. A. (1994). Personality dimensions and emotion systems. In P. Ekman & R. J. Davidson (Eds.), *The nature of emotion: Fundamental questions (Series in affective science)* (1st ed., pp. 329–331). Oxford University Press.

Gross, J. J. (2015). Emotion regulation: Current status and future prospects. *Psychological Inquiry, 26*(1), 1–26. https://doi.org/10.1080/1047840X.2014.940781

Hagger-Johnson, G., Roberts, B., Boniface, D., Sabia, S., Batty, G. D., Elbaz, A., Singh-Manoux, A., & Deary, I. J. (2012). Neuroticism and cardiovascular disease mortality: socioeconomic status modifies the risk in women (UK Health and Lifestyle Survey). *Psychosomatic Medicine, 74*(6), 596–603. https://doi.org/10.1097/PSY.0b013e31825c85ca

Hallion, L. S., Steinman, S. A., Tolin, D. F., & Diefenbach, G. J. (2018). Psychometric properties of the Difficulties in Emotion Regulation Scale (DERS) and its short forms in adults with emotional disorders. *Frontiers in Psychology, 9*, 539. https://doi.org/10.3389/fpsyg.2018.00539

Hamzah, S. R., Suandi, T., Ismail, M., & Muda, Z. (2019). Association of the personal factors of culture, attitude and motivation with health behavior among adolescents in Malaysia. *International Journal of Adolescence and Youth, 24*(2), 149–159. https://doi.org/10.1080/02673843.2018.1482772

Hayes, S. C., Wilson, K. G., Gifford, E. V., Follette, V. M., & Strosahl, K. (1996). Experiential avoidance and behavioral disorders: A functional dimensional approach to diagnosis and treatment. *Journal of Consulting and Clinical Psychology, 64*(6), 1152–1168. https://doi.org/10.1037/0022-006X.64.6.1152

Higgins, S. T. (2014). Behavior change, health, and health disparities: An introduction. *Preventive Medicine, 68*, 1–4. https://doi.org/10.1016/j.ypmed.2014.10.007

Hirani, K., Cherian, S., Mutch, R., & Payne, D. N. (2018). Identification of health risk behaviours among adolescent refugees resettling in Western Australia. *Archives of Disease in Childhood, 103*(3), 240–246. https://doi.org/10.1136/archdischild-2017-31345.

Houck, C. D., Barker, D. H., Hadley, W., Brown, L. K., Lansing, A., Almy, B., & Hancock, E. (2016). The 1-year impact of an emotion regulation intervention on early adolescent health risk behaviors. *Health Psychology: Official Journal of the Division of Health Psychology, American Psychological Association, 35*(9), 1036–1045. https://doi.org/10.1037/hea0000360

Jessor, R. (1991). Risk behavior in adolescence: A psychosocial framework for understanding and action. *The Journal of Adolescent Health: Official Publication of the Society for Adolescent Medicine, 12*(8), 597–605. https://doi.org/10.1016/1054-139X(91)90007-K

John, O. P., & Gross, J. J. (2004). Healthy and unhealthy emotion regulation: Personality processes, individual differences, and life span development. *Journal of Personality, 72*(6), 1301–1334. https://doi.org/10.1111/j.1467-6494.2004.00298.x

Johns, M. M., Lowry, R., Andrzejewski, J., Barrios, L. C., Demissie, Z., McManus, T., Rasberry, C. N., Robin, L., & Underwood, J. M. (2019). Transgender identity and experiences of violence victimization, substance use, suicide risk, and sexual risk behaviors among high school Students - 19 States and Large Urban School Districts, 2017. *MMWR. Morbidity and Mortality Weekly Report, 68*(3), 67–71. https://doi.org/10.15585/mmwr.mm6803a3

Kaplan, R. M. (2014). Behavior change and reducing health disparities. *Preventive Medicine, 68*, 5–10. https://doi.org/10.1016/j.ypmed.2014.04.014

Kokkonen, M., & Pulkkinen, L. (2001). Extraversion and neuroticism as antecedents of emotion regulation and dysregulation in adulthood. *European Journal of Personality, 15*(6), 407–424. https://doi.org/10.1002/per.425

Lansing, A. E., Plante, W. Y., Golshan, S., Fenemma-Notestine, C., & Thuret, S. (2019). Emotion regulation mediates the relationship between verbal learning and internalizing, trauma-related and externalizing symptoms among early-onset, persistently delinquent adolescents. *Learning and Individual Differences, 70*, 201–215. https://doi.org/10.1016/j.lindif.2017.01.014

Lee, A. M., Gurka, M. J., & DeBoer, M. D. (2016). Trends in metabolic syndrome severity and lifestyle factors among adolescents. *Pediatrics, 137*(3), e20153177. https://doi.org/10.1542/peds.2015-3177

Lima, C. A. G., Maia, M. D. F. M., Brito, M. F. S. F., Pinho, L. D., & Silveira, M. F. (2020). Psychometric properties of the Youth Risk Behavior Survey (YRBS) instrument in Brazilian college students. *Paidéia (Ribeirão Preto), 30*, e3006, 1–12. https://doi.org/10.1590/1982-4327e3006

Lozano-Madrid, M., Clark Bryan, D., Granero, R., Sánchez, I., Riesco, N., Mallorquí-Bagué, N., Jiménez-Murcia, S., Treasure, J., & Fernández-Aranda, F. (2020). Impulsivity, emotional dysregulation and executive function deficits could be associated with alcohol and drug abuse in eating disorders. *Journal of Clinical Medicine, 9*(6), 1936. https://doi.org/10.3390/jcm9061936

Malouff, J. M., Thorsteinsson, E. B., Rooke, S. E., & Schutte, N. S. (2007). Alcohol involvement and the five-factor model of personality: A meta-analysis. *Journal of Drug Education, 37*(3), 277–294. https://doi.org/10.2190/DE.37.3.d

Malouff, J. M., Thorsteinsson, E. B., & Schutte, N. S. (2005). The relationship between the five-factor model of personality and symptoms of clinical disorders: A meta-analysis. *Journal of Psychopathology and Behavioral Assessment, 27*(2), 101–114. https://doi.org/10.1007/s10862-005-5384-y

Malouff, J. M., Thorsteinsson, E. B., & Schutte, N. S. (2006). The five-factor model of personality and smoking: A meta-analysis. *Journal of Drug Education, 36*(1), 47–58. https://doi.org/10.2190/9EP8-17P8-EKG7-66AD

Mroczek, D. K., & Almeida, D. M. (2004). The effect of daily stress, personality, and age on daily negative affect. *Journal of Personality, 72*(2), 355–378. https://doi.org/10.1111/j.0022-3506.2004.00265.x

Murray, A. L., & Booth, T. (2015). Personality and physical health. *Current Opinion in Psychology, 5*, 50–55. https://doi.org/10.1016/j.copsyc.2015.03.011

Napier, A. D., Ancarno, C., Butler, B., Calabrese, J., Chater, A., Chatterjee, H., Guesnet, F., Horne, R., Jacyna, S., Jadhav, S., Macdonald, A., Neuendorf, U., Parkhurst, A., Reynolds, R., Scambler, G., Shamdasani, S., Smith, S. Z., Stougaard-Nielsen, J., Thomson, L., ... Woolf, K. (2014). Culture and health. *The Lancet, 384*(9954), 1607–1639. https://doi.org/10.1016/S0140-6736(14)61603-2

Preacher, K. J., & Hayes, A. F. (2004). SPSS and SAS procedures for estimating indirect effects in simple mediation models. *Behavior Research Methods, Instruments, & Computers: A Journal of the Psychonomic Society, Inc, 36*(4), 717–731. https://doi.org/10.3758/bf03206553

Preacher, K. J., & Hayes, A. F. (2008). Contemporary approaches to assessing mediation in communication research. In A. F. Hayes, M. D. Slater, & L. B. Snyder (Eds.), *The Sage sourcebook of advanced data analysis methods for communication research* (pp. 13–54). Sage Publications, Inc. https://doi.org/10.4135/9781452272054.n2

Purnamaningsih, E. H. (2017). Personality and emotion regulation strategies. *International Journal of Psychological Research, 10*(1), 53–60. https://doi.org/10.21500/20112084.2040

Raine, A., Dodge, K., Loeber, R., Gatzke-Kopp, L., Lynam, D., Reynolds, C., Stouthamer-Loeber, M., & Liu, J. (2006). The reactive–proactive aggression questionnaire: Differential correlates of reactive and proactive aggression in adolescent boys. *Aggressive Behavior, 32*(2), 159–171. https://doi.org/10.1002/ab.20115

Ram, D., George, M., & Gowdappa, B. (2018). Correlation of cognitive functions with emotional dysregulation in alcohol dependence: A preliminary study. *Indian Journal of Psychiatry, 60*(3), 307–311. https://doi.org/10.4103/psychiatry.IndianJPsychiatry_183_18

Sherry, S. B., Hewitt, P. L., Flett, G. L., Lee-Baggley, D. L., & Hall, P. A. (2007). Trait perfectionism and perfectionistic self-presentation in personality pathology. *Personality and Individual Differences, 42*(3), 477–490. https://doi.org/10.1016/j.paid.2006.07.026

Shipley, B. A., Weiss, A., Der, G., Taylor, M. D., & Deary, I. J. (2007). Neuroticism, extraversion, and mortality in the UK Health and Lifestyle Survey: A 21-year prospective cohort study. *Psychosomatic Medicine, 69*(9), 923–931. https://doi.org/10.1097/PSY.0b013e31815abf83

Smith, T. W. (2006). Personality as risk and resilience in physical health. *Current Directions in Psychological Science, 15*(5), 227–231. https://doi.org/10.1111/j.1467-8721.2006.00441.x

Smith, A. R., Chein, J., & Steinberg, L. (2014). Peers increase adolescent risk taking even when the probabilities of negative outcomes are known. *Developmental Psychology, 50*(5), 1564–1568. https://doi.org/10.1037/a0035696

Smith, T. W., & MacKenzie, J. (2006). Personality and risk of physical illness. *Annual Review of Clinical Psychology, 2*(1), 435–467. https://doi.org/10.1146/annurev.clinpsy.2.022305.095257

Steptoe, A. (2007). Health behaviour and stress. In G. Fink (Ed.), *Encyclopedia of stress* (2nd ed., pp. 263–266). Academic Press.

Suls, J., & Bunde, J. (2005). Anger, anxiety, and depression as risk factors for cardiovascular disease: The problems and implications of overlapping affective dispositions. *Psychological Bulletin, 131*(2), 260–300. https://doi.org/10.1037/0033-2909.131.2.260

Suls, J., Green, P., & Hillis, S. (1998). Emotional reactivity to everyday problems, affective inertia, and neuroticism. *Personality and Social Psychology Bulletin, 24*(2), 127–136. https://doi.org/10.1177/0146167298242002

Thompson, R. A. (1994). Emotion regulation: A theme in search of definition. *Monographs of the Society for Research in Child Development, 59*(2–3), 25–52. https://doi.org/10.1111/j.1540-5834.1994.tb01276.x

Trobst, K. K., Wiggins, J. S., Costa, P. T., Jr., Herbst, J. H., McCrae, R. R., & MastersIII, H. L. (2000). Personality psychology and problem behaviors: HIV risk and the five-factor model. *Journal of Personality, 68*(6), 1233–1252. https://doi.org/10.1111/1467-6494.00133

Turiano, N. A. (2012). *The health behavior model of personality (No. AAI3545444)*. ProQuest LLC. https://docs.lib.purdue.edu/dissertations/AAI3545444/

Turiano, N. A., Chapman, B. P., Gruenewald, T. L., & Mroczek, D. K. (2015). Personality and the leading behavioral contributors of mortality. *Health Psychology: Official Journal of the Division of Health Psychology, American Psychological Association, 34*(1), 51–60. https://doi.org/10.1037/hea0000038

Turiano, N. A., Mroczek, D. K., Moynihan, J., & Chapman, B. P. (2013). Big 5 personality traits and interleukin-6: Evidence for "healthy Neuroticism" in a US population sample. *Brain, Behavior, and Immunity, 28*, 83–89. https://doi.org/10.1016/j.bbi.2012.10.020

Turiano, N. A., Whiteman, S. D., Hampson, S. E., Roberts, B. W., & Mroczek, D. K. (2012). Personality and substance use in midlife: Conscientiousness as a moderator and the effects of trait change. *Journal of Research in Personality, 46*(3), 295–305. https://doi.org/10.1016/j.jrp.2012.02.009

Underwood, J. M., Brener, N., Thornton, J., Harris, W. A., Bryan, L. N., Shanklin, S. L., Deputy, N., Roberts, A. M., Queen, B., Chyen, D., Whittle, L., Lim, C., Yamakawa, Y., Leon-Nguyen, M., Kilmer, G., Smith-Grant, J., Demissie, Z., Jones, S. E., Clayton, H., & Dittus, P. (2020). Overview and methods for the youth risk behavior surveillance system - United States, 2019. *MMWR Supplements, 69*(1), 1–10. https://doi.org/10.15585/mmwr.su6901a1

van den Bos, W., & Hertwig, R. (2017). Adolescents display distinctive tolerance to ambiguity and to uncertainty during risky decision making. *Scientific Reports, 7*(1), 40962. https://doi.org/10.1038/srep40962

Vollrath, M., & Torgersen, S. (2002). Who takes health risks? A probe into eight personality types. *Personality and Individual Differences, 32*(7), 1185–1197. https://doi.org/10.1016/S0191-8869(01)00080-0

Vollrath, M., Torgersen, S., & Alnaes, R. (1995). Personality as long-term predictor of coping. *Personality and Individual Differences, 18*(1), 117–125. https://doi.org/10.1016/0191-8869(94)00110-E

Watson, D., & Clark, L. A. (1994). The vicissitudes of mood: A schematic model. In P. Ekman & R. J. Davidson (Eds.), *The nature of emotion: Fundamental questions (series in affective science).* (1st ed., pp. 400–405). Oxford University Press.

Watson, D., & Hubbard, B. (1996). Adaptational style and dispositional structure: Coping in the context of the five-factor model. *Journal of Personality, 64*(4), 737–774. https://doi.org/10.1111/j.1467-6494.1996.tb00943.x

Webb, T. L., Miles, E., & Sheeran, P. (2012). Dealing with feeling: A meta-analysis of the effectiveness of strategies derived from the process model of emotion regulation. *Psychological Bulletin, 138*(4), 775–808. https://doi.org/10.1037/a0027600

Weiss, H. A., & Ferrand, R. A. (2019). Improving adolescent health: An evidence-based call to action. *The Lancet, 393*(10176), 1073–1075. https://doi.org/10.1016/S0140-6736(18)32996-9

Weiss, N. H., Sullivan, T. P., & Tull, M. T. (2015). Explicating the role of emotion dysregulation in risky behaviors: A review and synthesis of the literature with directions for future research and clinical practice. *Current Opinion in Psychology, 3*, 22–29. https://doi.org/10.1016/j.copsyc.2015.01.013

Weston, S. J., Hill, P. L., Edmonds, G. W., Mroczek, D. K., & Hampson, S. E. (2019). No Evidence of "healthy neuroticism" in the Hawaii Personality and Health Cohort. *Annals of Behavioral Medicine : a Publication of the Society of Behavioral Medicine, 53*(5), 426–441. https://doi.org/10.1093/abm/kay055

Weston, S. J., & Jackson, J. J. (2015). Identification of the healthy neurotic: Personality traits predict smoking after disease onset. *Journal of Research in Personality, 54*, 61–69. https://doi.org/10.1016/j.jrp.2014.04.008

Weston, S. J., & Jackson, J. J. (2016). How do people respond to health news? The role of personality traits. *Psychology & Health, 31*(6), 637–654. https://doi.org/10.1080/08870446.2015.1119274

World Health Organization. (2015). *Global Strategy for Women's, Children's and Adolescent's Health 2016-2030*. WHO. https://www.who.int/life-course/partners/global-strategy/globalstrategyreport2016-2030-lowres.pdf.

World Health Organization. (2021). Adolescent and young adult health. https://www.who.int/en/news-room/fact-sheets/detail/adolescents-health-risks-and-solutions

Zafar, H., Debowska, A., & Boduszek, D. (2021). Emotion regulation difficulties and psychopathology among Pakistani adolescents. *Clinical Child Psychology and Psychiatry, 26*(1), 121–139. https://doi.org/10.1177/1359104520969765

Zimmermann, K. S., Richardson, R., & Baker, K. D. (2019). Maturational changes in prefrontal and amygdala circuits in adolescence: Implications for understanding fear inhibition during a vulnerable period of development. *Brain Sciences, 9*(3), 65. https://doi.org/10.3390/brainsci9030065

How Compassionate Abilities Influence the Experience of Loneliness and Quality of Life of People with and without Chronic Physical Disease?

Tânia Ramalho, Joana Pereira and Cláudia Ferreira

ABSTRACT

The current study aimed to test whether individuals with and without a chronic physical disease differ in levels of compassionate abilities, loneliness and quality of life (QoL); and to examine whether loneliness mediated the impact of self-compassion and of receiving compassion from others in physical, psychological, and social QoL. In this cross-sectional study, individuals with ($n = 278$) and without ($n = 455$) physical chronic disease were recruited through an online self-report protocol. The Compassionate Attributes and Engagement Scale, the UCLA Loneliness Scale, and the World Health Organization's QoL-BREF were used. Individuals with a chronic physical disease diagnosis reported lower compassionate abilities and QoL, as well as higher levels of loneliness, when compared to participants without a diagnosis. For both samples, compassionate abilities were negatively linked to loneliness, and positively linked to QoL. Path analysis results indicated that compassionate abilities have a direct effect on loneliness, which explains individuals' perceived QoL. Results highlight the crucial role of self-compassion skills and the ability to perceive others as compassionate, in loneliness and QoL, both in individuals with and without a chronic physical disease. These findings seem to have important research and clinical implications.

As societies have improved their living conditions, health habits, medical knowledge and practice, there has been an increase in life expectancy (Niccoli & Partridge, 2012; Ribeiro et al., 2017). This improvement in life expectancy and healthcare systems has been associated with an exponential increase in chronic disease. Approximately 50% of the population in the United States (US) has been diagnosed with, at least, one chronic disease (Ward & Schiller, 2013). In Europe, it is estimated that over 50 million citizens suffer from multiple chronic conditions (Heide et al., 2015). In Portugal, according to Romana et al. (2019), 57.8% of the population between 25 and 74 years of age have been diagnosed with one or more chronic disease. Even though the definition of chronic disease is not consensual, most studies define it based on its prolonged duration (at least six months), poor prognosis (uncertain or no cure), pattern of reoccurrence and deterioration, and its consequences, that cause sequelae on an individual's quality of life (QoL) (O'Halloran et al., 2004).

Research has shown a growing interest in exploring both the impact of chronic disease on QoL and the strategies that can promote well-being in these patients (McIntyre et al., 2019; Ribeiro et al., 2017). According to the World Health Organization (WHO), QoL can be defined as "a person's perception of his/her position in life within the context of the culture and value systems in which he/she lives and in relation to his/her goals, expectations, standards, and concerns" (WHOQOL Group, 1994, p. 28). This conceptualization of QoL takes into account physical, psychological, social, and environmental variables, such as the quality of relationships (WHOQOL Group, 1994). Therefore, it is important to explore the impact of potential risk and protective factors on the specific domains of QoL, namely in its psychological, physical, and social domains.

The importance of compassion in literature has risen in the last few decades (Gilbert et al., 2017). Although compassion has many different definitions, Gilbert defines it as the capacity to empathize with the suffering of the self and others (compassionate engagement), and to act to reduce and prevent suffering (compassionate actions) (Gilbert, 2017; Gilbert & Choden, 2013). Furthermore, Gilbert et al. (2017) argue that in compassion it is possible to identify three flows: (*i*) one directed toward the self (self-compassion), *(ii)* another directed toward others (compassion for others) and finally *(iii)* one directed from others (compassion from others), i.e. perceiving and being open to receive gestures of care, support and compassion toward us.

One of the processes that has been linked to QoL is self-compassion (e.g. Bohadana et al., 2019), both in chronically ill and in healthy individuals (Dowd & Jung, 2017; Finlay-Jones et al., 2020; Pinto-Gouveia et al., 2014; Sirois & Hirsch, 2019). According to recent studies, self-compassion can have a positive impact on QoL through different mechanisms, either by promoting adherence to treatments and diets or attenuating psychopathological symptoms and negative experiences (Dowd & Jung, 2017; Pinto-Gouveia et al., 2014; Sirois & Hirsch, 2019). A growing body of research has suggested that self-compassion can have a protective role in mental health and QoL, especially when individuals face challenging life circumstances, such as a life-threatening disease or a chronic condition (e.g. Hlabangana & Hearn, 2020; Pinto-Gouveia et al., 2014).

Beyond being associated with a series of positive indicators, such as happiness (e.g. Wollast et al., 2019) and QoL (Itzick et al., 2018), research has shown that self-compassion is negatively associated with indicators of poor psychological adjustment (e.g. Hermanto et al., 2016), such as loneliness (Akin, 2010; Itzick et al., 2018; Lyon, 2015). Nonetheless, studies that have explored the relationship between compassion and loneliness are limited, since they have only focused on self-compassion, compassion satisfaction or compassion fatigue and have excluded the exploration of the relationship between loneliness and other flows of compassion. In spite of this, it is theoretically expected that the ability to be open to receiving gestures of care and support and experiencing others as more compassionate (compassion from others) may be associated with decreased loneliness.

Loneliness can be characterized as the negative subjective experience that individuals go through when they perceive that their social relationships are not fulfilling their emotional needs (Perlman & Peplau, 1982). Also, it is important to point out that there are differences between loneliness and social isolation (Cacioppo et al., 2015; Russell et al., 2012). Perceiving higher levels of loneliness does not mean that the person is indeed physically alone (e.g. Hawkley & Cacioppo, 2010). The individual can be isolated but not feel lonely, or experiences loneliness despite being surrounded by people (Cacioppo et al., 2015; Perlman & Peplau, 1982). Therefore, the perception of being on their own, of not being understood, or of not belonging leads to experiences of loneliness (Cacioppo et al., 2015; Rokach, 2012; Russell et al., 1984).

Loneliness has been considered one of the most relevant issues of public health (Leigh-Hunt et al., 2017), mainly due to its link with various indicators. These indicators may be physical (such as blood pressure levels and immune response; Hawkley et al., 2010; Pressman et al., 2005) or psychological (such as anxiety and depressive symptoms, and suicidal ideation; Beutel et al., 2017; Hyland et al., 2019; McClelland et al., 2020), but also be indicators of premature mortality (e.g. Holt-Lunstad et al., 2010) or a lower QoL (e.g. Arslantaş et al., 2015; Hyland et al., 2019; Tan et al., 2020). Literature suggests that the study of loneliness is particularly relevant in chronically ill individuals (Stickley & Koyanagi, 2018). Indeed, when experiencing loneliness, individuals with chronic disease tend to have a more negative perception of their condition, of the severity of their symptoms, and a lower perception of the efficacy of the treatment. In turn, this leads to negative emotions and deterioration of physical and mental health (Dong et al., 2012; Özkan Tuncay et al., 2018). Furthermore, individuals who experience loneliness tend to have implicit hypervigilance to negative social interactions, leading them to behave accordingly (Newall et al., 2009). Ultimately, this behavior tends to increase their levels of loneliness and may explain lower satisfaction in their social relationships (Newall et al., 2009).

Even though there is growing evidence on loneliness as an important upstream factor which has an impact on well-being, its relationship with the ability to receive compassion (both from the self and others) and the way it affects different domains of QoL (physical, psychological, and social domains) have not clearly and specifically been studied before. The current study aimed to fill this gap so that more effective interventions can be developed to reduce the experience of loneliness and its harmful impact on well-being (Stickley et al., 2015). Therefore, the aims of the present study were: 1) to test whether individuals with and without a chronic physical disease differ in levels of compassion, loneliness, and QoL (in its physical, psychological and social domains); and 2) to test a model to explore whether the abilities to receive compassion (from the self and others) influence loneliness and have an impact on QoL (in its core domains), while controlling for the effect of age. Additionally, the plausibility of the model was tested taking into account two groups (with and without a chronic physical disease). It was hypothesized that compassionate abilities may be associated with lower experiences of loneliness and better physical, psychological, and social QoL, and that loneliness would have a mediation role in this relationship.

Material and Methods

Participants

The study sample consisted of 733 participants that comprised two groups: (1) participants who reported a clinical diagnosis of chronic physical disease and (2) participants who did not report a clinical diagnosis of chronic physical disease.

The group of individuals diagnosed with a physical chronic disease was comprised of 278 participants (37.9%). This group was mostly composed of women ($n = 238$; 85.6%), presented a mean age of 42.20 years ($SD = 12.17$) and a mean of 13.51 ($SD = 3.20$) years of education. Most of the participants were currently married/living with a partner ($n = 147$; 52.9%), employed ($n = 167$; 60.1%), and living in an urban area ($n = 150$; 54%). Time since diagnosis varied between 1 and 684 months ($M = 145.38$; $SD = 138.69$). The majority had not attended psychological or psychiatric consultations ($n = 200$; 71.9%). Table 1 presents the distribution of physical chronic diseases reported by participants.

The group in which a physical chronic disease was not reported was comprised of 455 participants (62.1%), 327 women (71.9%), with mean age of 31.73 ($SD = 12.10$) years and a mean of 14.03 ($SD = 2.75$) years of education. Most participants were single ($n = 283$; 62.2%), currently employed ($n = 256$; 56.3%), and living in an urban area ($n = 189$; 41.5%). The majority had not attended psychological or psychiatric consultations ($n = 402$; 88.4%). Significant differences were found between the participants from the groups with and without a diagnosis of physical chronic disease regarding social demographic variables: gender [$\chi^2_{(1)} = 18.45$; $p < .001$; Cramer's $V = .16$], age [$t_{(731)} = -11.35$; $p < .001$; Cohen's $d = .86$], marital status [$\chi^2_{(3)} = 71.40$; $p < .001$; Cramer's $V = .31$], professional situation [$\chi^2_{(4)} = 100.99$; $p < .001$; Cramer's $V = .37$], area of residence [$\chi^2_{(2)} = 12.89$; $p = .002$; Cramer's $V = .13$], years of education [$t_{(519.049)} = 2.24$; $p = .025$; Cohen's $d = .17$].

Procedures

This cross-sectional study is part of broader research that aims to understand the role of compassionate abilities, loneliness, and perceived QoL in physical chronic disease patients. This study was approved by the Ethical Committee of the Faculty of Psychology and Educational Science of the University of Coimbra.

The recruitment of the participants for the study occurred between October 2019 and January 2020. Participants were electronically invited to participate in the research *via* email (e.g. institutions related to chronic disease) and social media websites (e.g. Facebook, Instagram). The invitation included information about the purpose of the study, its procedures and voluntary nature, the confidentiality of the data, and a link, which directed eventual participants to the online version of the research protocol. Participants that agreed to take part gave their informed consent and completed the research protocol within approximately 20 min. Participants were asked if they had, or

Table 1. Chronic Diseases Reported by Participants.

Disease	*N*	%
Autoimmune (e.g. Lupus disease)	87	23.8
Neuromuscular (e.g. Fibromyalgia)	83	22.7
Gastrointestinal (e.g. Crohn's disease)	54	14.8
Dermatological (e.g. Suppurative Hidradenitis)	40	10.9
Respiratory (e.g. asthma)	33	9.0
Cardiovascular (e.g. diabetes)	19	5.2
Oncological (e.g. breast cancer)	16	4.4
Others	34	9.3

did not have, one or more diagnoses of chronic physical disease. For those who answered positively, questions about their disease were then presented (e.g. type of disease, time of diagnosis). A total of 818 participants completed the protocol. The eligibility criteria to participate in the study were: (1) to be aged between eighteen and sixty-five; (2) to be a resident in Portugal; and (3) to be a native speaker of Portuguese. Considering the inclusion criteria, 85 participants were excluded from the analyses: 36 who were younger than 18 or older than 65; 47 who did not live in Portugal, and 2 who did not identify their chronic physical disease. There were no missing data because participants had to answer all the items in order to be able to submit the protocol.

Measures

Participants were asked about their demographic data (e.g. gender, age, years of education, area of residence, marital status, and professional situation) and medical data (e.g. if they had been diagnosed with a chronic physical disease, the type of disease they had been diagnosed with, and time since their diagnosis). Participants completed the validated Portuguese versions of the following measures:

The Compassionate Attributes and Engagement Scales (CEAS, original and Portuguese version: Gilbert et al., 2017). CEAS is a self-report instrument to measure compassion that comprises three separate scales to assess its three flows: self-compassion (e.g. "I am motivated to engage and work with my distress when it arises."), compassion toward others (e.g. "I notice and am sensitive to distress in others when it arises") and compassion received from others (e.g. "Others direct their attention to what is likely to be helpful to me"). Each scale consists of 13 items and assesses a person's compassionate attributes (8 items) and compassionate actions (5 items) when suffering or facing difficult experiences. The items are answered on a 10-point scale ranging from 1 (*never*) to 10 (*always*), with higher scores indicating higher levels of openness to give or receive compassion. For this study, only the scale of self-compassion and that of compassion received from others were analyzed, which had both presented a good internal consistency in the original study (engagement α = .47; .89 and actions α = .90; .91, respectively; Gilbert et al., 2017). In the current protocol, Cronbach's alpha presented suitable values both in the group without a diagnosis of a physical chronic disease and in the group with a diagnosis of this type: self-compassion scale (engagement α = .81; .83; and actions α = .92; .92) and compassion from others scale (engagement α = .92; .94; and actions α = .95; .94), respectively.

The UCLA Loneliness Scale (UCLA LS-3; Russell, 1996; Portuguese version: Zeas-Sigüenza et al., 2020). UCLA LS-3 is composed of 20 items that assess the subjective perception of an individual's loneliness (e.g. "How often do you feel that you are "in tune" with the people around you?", "How often do you feel that you lack companionship?"). Participants are asked to rate each sentence using a 4-point scale, from 1 (*never*) to 4 (*often*), with higher scores indicating more prominent experiences of loneliness. Both the original study and the Portuguese validation of the UCLA LS-3 presented a good internal consistency (the original study conveyed Cronbach's alphas ranging from .89 to .94, across different samples, and the Portuguese version reported a α = .91). In this study, the Cronbach's alpha value was .92 for both groups.

The World Health Organization Quality of Life BREF (WHOQOL-BREF, WHOQOL Group, 1998; Portuguese version: Canavarro et al., 2007). The WHOQOL-BREF is a short self-report questionnaire developed by the World Health Organization and designed to assess the perception of quality of life (QoL). WHOQOL-BREF comprises 26 items, divided into four domains of QoL: physical, psychological, social, and environmental. Items are rated on a 5-point scale (ranging from 0 - "*Very dissatisfied*" to 5 – "*Very satisfied*"). All domain scores are transformed to reflect a 0 to 100 scale. Higher scores correspond to a better QoL. For this study, the Physical, Psychological, and Social domains were considered. The Cronbach's alpha in the original study ranged from .66 (Social) to .82 (Physical), and in the Portuguese version it ranged from .64 (Social) to .87 (Physical), representing an adequate internal consistency. In this study, Cronbach's alpha ranged from .74 (Social) to .84 (Psychological) in the group without a diagnosis of a physical chronic disease and from .77 (Social) to .85 (Psychological) in the group with a diagnosis of this type.

Statistical Analyses

Descriptive statistics (means, standard deviations (*SD*) and frequencies), comparison tests (*t*-tests and qui-square tests), and correlation analyses were conducted using the IBM SPSS Statistics 22.0 software (SPSS IBM; Chicago, IL). Pearson product-moment correlations analyses were performed to explore the association between Self-compassion (CEAS_SC), compassion from others (CEAS_FROM), loneliness (UCLA), physical QoL (QoL_Physical), psychological QoL (QoL_Psy), social QoL (QoL_Social), and age. Effect sizes of the correlations were analyzed according to recommended guidelines (Cohen et al., 2003): small: r = .10 to .29; moderate: r = .30 to .49; large: r = .50 to .69; very large: r = .70 to .89; nearly perfect: $r \geq .90$; and perfect: $r = 1$. Student's t-test and χ^2 test were conducted to analyze the differences between the two populations. The correlation magnitude was calculated using Cramer's V for χ^2 test and with Cohen's d for Student's t-test. The results were interpreted based on the recommendations of Cohen (1992): small: $d \geq .20$, Cramer's $V \geq .01$; medium: $d \geq .50$, Cramer's $V \geq .03$; large: $d \geq .80$, Cramer's $V \geq .05$.

Finally, the AMOS software (version 22 Arbuckle, 2013) was used to examine the proposed model (Figure 1), which tested the hypothesis that self-compassion and compassion from others (exogenous independent variables) would present a significant effect on QoL (physical, psychological, and social relationship; endogenous dependent variables), through the mediational effects of loneliness (endogenous, mediator variable), while controlling the effect of age. The Maximum Likelihood method was performed with the aim of test regression coefficients and computing fit statistics. Additionally, a group of goodness-of-fit indices, such as Chi square ($\chi 2$; $p > .05$), normed Chi square (CMIN/df < 5), Tucker-Lewis Index (TLI > .95), Comparative Fit Index (CFI > .95), and the Root Mean Square Error of Approximation index (RMSEA < .08), were examined to ensure the adequacy of the overall model (Hu & Bentler, 1999). Furthermore, through the Bootstrap resampling method, the significance of the

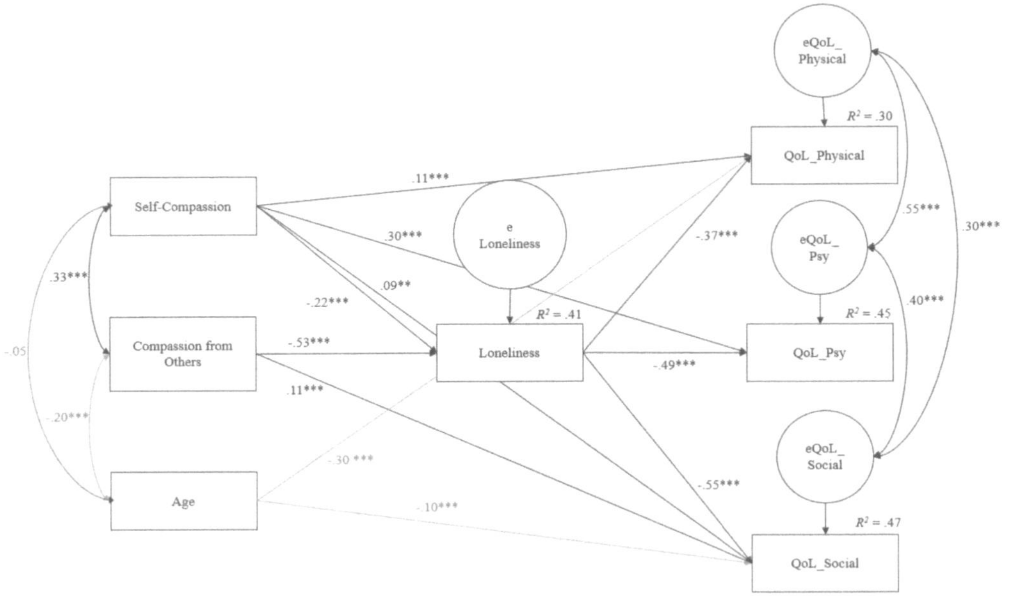

Figure 1. Final path model.*Note.* QoL_Physical = Physical Quality of Life; QoL_Psy = Psychological Quality of Life; QoL_Social = Social Quality of Life.R^2 = square multiple correlations; e = the measurement errors; * $p < .05$; ** $p < .01$; *** $p < .001$

paths was analyzed, with 5000 Bootstrap samples, and 95% bias-corrected confidence intervals around the standardizer estimates of total, direct, and indirect effects. For the effect to be statistically significant ($p < .05$), the confidence interval cannot contain the value zero in it. Finally, the invariance of the model was examined across the individuals with ($n = 278$) and without ($n = 455$) physical chronic disease. Two models were considered: an unconstrained model, testing if the structure of the model was invariant, with no measurement parameters constrained to be equal; and, a measurement weights model (model loadings constrained to be equal). When the added restriction did not lead to a worse model fit, it was considered invariant. Given that the χ^2 difference test is highly sensitive to sample size, statistical differences between models were assessed through the difference between Comparative Fit Indices (ΔCFI), where a value equal to or lower than .01 indicates strong invariance (Cheung & Rensvold, 2002).

Results

Preliminary Analyses

The assumption of the normality of the variables' distribution was verified by the analysis of Skewness and Kurtosis' values (Kline, 2005). Preliminary analyses demonstrated that data followed the assumptions of normality, linearity, homoscedasticity, multicollinearity, independence of errors and singularity among the variables, which indicates suitability for regression analyses (Field, 2004).

Differences in the Study Variables

As Table 2 shows, the group of participants diagnosed with a chronic physical disease reported lower levels of self-compassion, lower ability to receive compassion from others and decreased QoL (physical, psychological, and social relationships), and higher levels of loneliness, compared with group in which participants did not have a diagnosis.

Correlation Analyses

Results from correlation analyses are reported in Table 3. In both groups, significant and positive associations were found between self-compassion and compassion from others, physical QoL, psychological QoL, and social QoL, and significant negative associations were found between self-compassion and loneliness. Receiving compassion from others was significantly and positively associated with physical QoL, psychological QoL, and social QoL, and significantly and negatively associated with loneliness in both groups. Significant and negative associations were found between loneliness, physical QoL, psychological QoL, and social QoL in both groups. Physical QoL was significantly positively associated with psychological QoL and social QoL in both groups. Psychological QoL was significantly and positively associated with social QoL, in both groups. Significant and negative associations were found between age and receiving compassion from others and physical QoL and significant positive

Table 2. Means (M), Standard Deviation (SD) and Comparison Between Participants With ($n = 278$) and Without a Physical Chronic Disease Diagnosis ($n = 455$).

	Participants with a Physical Chronic Disease diagnosis	Participants without a Physical Chronic Disease diagnosis			
	M (SD)	*M (SD)*	*t*	*p*	*d*
Self-compassion	76.00 (16.45)	78.70 (16.33)	2.17	**.030**	.16
Compassion from Others	66.21 (21.72)	75.85 (19.73)	6.04	**<.001**	.47
Loneliness	48.20 (10.42)	43.31 (9.43)	−6.55	**<.001**	.49
QoL_Physical	48.00 (19.34)	73.55 (15.11)	18.80	**<.001**	1.47
QoL_Psy	55.47 (19.82)	67.60 (16.15)	8.61	**<.001**	.67
QoL_Social	52.37 (23.77)	67.51 (19.58)	8.93	**<.001**	.70

Notes. QoL_Physical = Physical Quality of Life; QoL_Psy = Psychological Quality of Life; QoL_Social = Social Quality of Life.

Table 3. Correlations among the Study Variables.

	1	2	3	4	5	6	7
1.Self-compassion	–	**.27*** **	**-.36*** **	**.21*** **	**.52*** **	**.36*** **	**.08**
2.Compassion from others	.37***	–	**-.62*** **	**.31*** **	**.37*** **	**.47*** **	**-.10**
3.Loneliness	-.41***	-.55***	–	**-.36*** **	**-.58*** **	**-.66*** **	**.05**
4.QoL_Physical	.34***	.23***	-.44***	–	**.57*** **	**.40*** **	**-.15** **
5.QoL_Psy	.50***	.31***	-.58***	.62***	–	**.64*** **	**.05**
6.QoL_Social	.34***	.44***	-.63***	.46***	.58***	–	**-.07**
7.Age	-.07	-.15**	.03	-.14**	.10*	-.06	–

Notes. The values that are **in bold** are refer to the with diagnosis of physical chronic disease group ($n = 278$) and the ones who are below are from the without diagnosis group ($n = 455$).
QoL_Physical = Physical Quality of Life; QoL_Psy = Psychological Quality of Life; QoL_Social = Social Quality of Life.
* $p < .05$; ** $p < .01$; *** $p < .001$.

associations with psychological QoL, in the group in which participants did not have a physical chronic disease. In the group diagnosed with a diagnosis of this type, age was significantly and negatively associated with physical QoL.

Path Analysis

A path analysis was executed in order to test whether loneliness (UCLA) mediates the impact of self-compassion (CEAS_SC) and compassion from others (CEAS_FROM) on QoL (physical, psychological and social), by controlling the age. Initially, we tested the path model in a fully saturated model (with zero degrees of freedom) consisting of 35 parameters. Results showed that four paths were not significant: the direct effect of receiving compassion from others on psychological QoL ($b_{CEAS\_FROM} = -.01$; $SE_b = .03$; $Z = -.35$; $p = .724$); the direct effect of age on loneliness ($b_{AGE} = .01$; $SE_b = .02$; $Z = 0.37$; $p = .714$); the direct effect of age on psychological QoL ($b_{AGE} = .03$; $SE_b = .04$; $Z = .84$; $p = .400$); and the direct effect of receiving compassion from others on physical QoL ($b_{CEAS\_FROM} = .04$; $SE_b = .03$; $Z = 1.18$; $p = .237$). In order to have only significant paths, these paths were progressively deleted, and the model was readjusted.

The final model demonstrated an excellent fit to the empirical data, as suggested by the analysis of well-known and recommended goodness of fit indices [$\chi^2_{(4)} = 2.366$, $p = .669$, CMIN/DF = 0.592; TLI = 1.00; CFI = 1.000; RMSEA = 0.000, $p = .973$; 95% CI = .00 to .04], (Kline, 2005).

Analysis of Direct Effects

The analysis of the direct effects showed that self-compassion had a significant direct effect of −.22 on loneliness ($b_{CEAS\_SC} = -.14$; $SE_b = .02$; $Z = -7.37$; $p < .001$), of .11 on physical QoL ($b_{CEAS\_SC} = .14$; $SE_b = .04$; $Z = 3.18$; $p = .001$), of .30 on psychological QoL ($b_{CEAS\_SC} = .34$; $SE_b = .03$; $Z = 10.05$; $p < .001$), and of .09 on social QoL ($b_{CEAS\_SC} = .12$; $SE_b = .04$; $Z = 2.99$; $p = .003$). Moreover, receiving compassion from others had a direct effect of −.53 on loneliness ($b_{CEAS\_FROM} = -.25$; $SE_b = .02$; $Z = -17.41$; $p < .001$) and .11 on social QoL ($b_{CEAS\_FROM} = .12$; $SE_b = .03$; $Z = 3.46$; $p < .001$). Loneliness had a direct effect of −.37 on physical QoL ($b_{UCLA} = -.78$; $SE_b = .07$; $Z = -11.00$; $p < .001$), of −.49 on psychological QoL ($b_{UCLA} = -.90$; $SE_b = .06$; $Z = -16.30$; $p < .001$), and of −.55 on social QoL ($b_{UCLA} = -1.23$; $SE_b = .08$; $Z = -16.25$; $p < .001$). Lastly, age had a direct effect of −.30 on physical QoL ($b_{AGE} = -.48$; $SE_b = .04$; $Z = -11.49$; $p < .001$) and of −.10 on social QoL ($b_{AGE} = -.17$; $SE_b = .04$; $Z = -3.93$; $p < .001$).

Analysis of Indirect Effects

The analysis of the indirect effects showed that receiving compassion from others had an indirect effect of .20 (95% CI = .16/.24) on physical QoL, of .26 (95% CI = .22/.30), on psychological QoL, and of .29 (95% CI = .25/.34) on social QoL, through loneliness. Also, self-compassion had and indirect effect of .08 (95% CI = .06/.11) on physical QoL, of .11 (95% CI = .08/.14) on psychological QoL, and of .12 (95% CI = .09/.16) on social QoL, through loneliness.

The model explained 30% of the variance of physical QoL, 45% of psychological QoL, 47% of social QoL, and 41% of the variance of loneliness. All path coefficients were statistically significant ($p < .05$).

Finally, the invariance of this model was examined across the two groups (with a diagnosis of physical chronic disease group vs. without a diagnosis group) through a multigroup analysis. Results showed that the groups did not present significant differences [$\chi^2_{(11)} = 13.94$, $p = .236$]. As Table 4 shows, the results from the chi-square difference test between the unconstrained and the constrained models revealed that the model was invariant across the two groups that is, the groups did not present significant differences at the model level.

Discussion

The present study aimed to test whether individuals with and without a chronic physical disease differ in levels of compassion, loneliness, and QoL (in its physical, psychological and social domains). Additionally, this study aimed to test an integrative model that explored the effect of compassionate abilities on the physical, psychological, and social domains of QoL and the mediating role of loneliness in these associations. The model invariance across the individuals with and without a diagnosis of physical chronic disease was also tested.

Concerning the first aim of the study, the results are in line with literature by showing that individuals diagnosed with a physical chronic disease tend to report lower levels of self-compassion (e.g. Pinto-Gouveia et al., 2014) and of receiving compassion from others (Trindade et al., 2018), and higher levels of loneliness (e.g. Arslantaş et al., 2015), when compared with individuals that do not present a diagnosis. Moreover, these results corroborated previous research (e.g. Kilian et al., 2001) by showing that individuals who had been diagnosed with a physical chronic disease presented lower levels of perceived QoL (physical, psychological, and social domains) when compared to individuals without a diagnosis.

Correlational results were consistent with previous research indicating that both self-compassion and receiving compassion from others were negatively linked with loneliness (Akin, 2010; Lyon, 2015). This, in turn, was negatively linked with perceived QoL (e.g. Arslantaş et al., 2015; Tan et al., 2020). Additionally, and also according to prior literature, self-compassion, and receiving compassion from others were positively

Table 4. Results of the Multi-Group Analysis across the Unconstrained Model and the Constrained Models (Testing sample: $n = 455$; Validation Sample: $n = 455$).

	χ^2	*df*	CFI	RMSEA [95% CI]	$\Delta\chi^2$	Δdf	*p*	ΔCFI
Multi-group analyses								
Unconstrained model	24.62*	8	.990	.05 [.03-.08]				
Measurement weights	38.56*	19	.989	.04 [.02-.06]	182.04	7	**	.001

Note. χ2 = Chi-square goodness-of-fit statistic; *df* = degrees of freedom; CFI = comparative fit index; RMSEA = Root Mean Square Error of Approximation.
*χ^2 significant at $p < .05$.

associated with the domains of QoL (e.g. Hlabangana & Hearn, 2020; Pinto-Gouveia et al., 2014). These associations were observed in both groups.

To better understand the relationship between the study variables, a theoretical model was tested to explore the effect of compassionate abilities (self-compassion and receiving compassion from others) on the physical, psychological, and social domains of QoL, considering the role of loneliness, while controlling the effect of age in the all sample. Path analysis' findings indicated that the tested model showed an excellent fit to the empirical data, accounting for 30 per cent of the variance of physical QoL, 45 per cent of psychological QoL, and 47 per cent of social QoL. Furthermore, this model revealed that 41 per cent of the variance of loneliness was explained by self-compassionate abilities and by receiving compassion from others. Particularly, results showed that self-compassion has a direct effect on physical, psychological, and social QoL, and an indirect effect mediated by loneliness. Also, receiving compassion from others presented a direct effect on social domain of QoL and an indirect effect, through loneliness, on all QoL domains in study. A multigroup analysis revealed that the model was invariant across the individuals, with and without a diagnosis of physical chronic disease, suggesting that the relationships previously found between the variables occur in a similar way for both groups.

Overall results revealed that lower abilities to give ourselves gestures of care, support, and compassion, and to perceive others as compassionate toward us, explained the decrease of perceived physical, psychological, and social QoL, *via* higher levels of loneliness, even when controlling the effect of age. The study's findings add to current knowledge by emphasizing the role of compassionate abilities in loneliness (i.e. a subjective perception of social disconnectedness or a feeling of not belonging; Cacioppo et al., 2015; Russell et al., 1984), and clarifying the influence of this painful emotion on perceived QoL.

To our knowledge, this is the first study to focus on the relationship between compassionate abilities, loneliness and QoL (in its physical, psychological, and social domains) and to explore the role of receiving compassion both from the self and from others in individuals with and without a physical chronic disease diagnosis. In fact, previous literature has mainly focused on the study of the relationship between self-compassion (Akin, 2010; Dowd & Jung, 2017; Finlay-Jones et al., 2020; Lyon, 2015; Pinto-Gouveia et al., 2014; Sirois & Hirsch, 2019), compassion satisfaction or compassion fatigue (Itzick et al., 2018) with loneliness and QoL. Further, these findings arise as another step in research about the effect of loneliness on perceived QoL, which is still limited (e.g. Arslantaş et al., 2015; Tan et al., 2020). Finally, this study's sample, which includes a wide age range, contrasts with previous research that has evaluated feelings of loneliness in younger (Akin, 2010; Lyon, 2015; Shovestul et al., 2020) or older ages (Arslantaş et al., 2015; Schrempft et al., 2019; Tan et al., 2020).

Several limitations should be taken into consideration while interpreting our findings. First, although the directional paths tested in the analyses were grounded in previous research, the cross-sectional design nature of this study does not allow for causal conclusions. A longitudinal methodology should be privileged in future studies. Second, the current study used a self-report online protocol, which provided a larger sample, although it can produce sample bias, namely because only individuals with access to the Internet were able to participate. Additionally, the group of participants with a chronic physical disease was composed of diverse diagnoses, which may have different impacts on the individuals' lives. Future research should examine these associations among a specific diagnosis group. Moreover, the groups used in this study have significant sociodemographic differences, which should be considered in further investigations. The present model can, in the future, be enriched with different emotional regulation processes. Lastly, it should be noted that the model was tested within two groups of adults (with and without a chronic health condition) from the Portuguese population. Therefore the generalization of the study's findings to other cultures is limited. Future research should explore the proposed model in different countries and test its cross-culture invariance.

This study also has important implications for practice and research related to preventive intervention. These results highlight the need to evaluate loneliness in chronic physical disease. Specifically, this study underscores the important role of the ability of giving ourselves gestures of care, support, and compassion, and of receiving them from others in reducing an individual's perception of not being understood, or not belonging, which may explain individuals' perceived QoL. In this sense, data appears to suggest that programmes that aim to improve compassionate abilities targeting loneliness and QoL should be prioritized, especially for physical chronically ill individuals, given their specific requirements.

Acknowledgements

We thank all the participants who completed our protocol. We are grateful to Joana Castro and Sara Oliveira for their assistance in the construction of the present study.

Disclosure of Interest

The authors report no conflict of interest.

Data Availability Statement

The data that support the findings of this study are available from the corresponding author, Joana Pereira, upon reasonable request.

ORCID

Tânia Ramalho http://orcid.org/0000-0002-8970-3540
Joana Pereira http://orcid.org/0000-0001-7790-0830
Cláudia Ferreira http://orcid.org/0000-0002-7020-9606

References

Akin, A. (2010). Self-compassion and loneliness. *International Online Journal of Educational Sciences*, *2*(3), 702–718.

Arbuckle, J. L. (2013). Amos (Version 22.0). [Computer program]. IBM SPSS.

Arslantaş, H., Adana, F., Ergin, F. A., Kayar, D., & Acar, G. (2015). Loneliness in elderly people, associated factors, and its correlation with quality of life: A field study from western Turkey. *Iran Journal of Public Health*, *44*(1), 43–50. http://ijph.tums.ac.ir

Beutel, M. E., Klein, E. M., Brähler, E., Reiner, I., Jünger, C., Michal, M., Wiltink, J., Wild, P. S., Münzel, T., Lackner, K. J., & Tibubos, A. N. (2017). Loneliness in the general population: Prevalence, determinants and relations to mental health. *BioMed Central Psychiatry*, *17*(97). https://doi.org/10.1186/s12888-017-1262-x

Bohadana, G., Morrissey, S., & Paynter, J. (2019). Self-compassion: A novel predictor of stress and quality of life in parents of children with autism spectrum disorder. *Journal of Autism and Developmental Disorders*, *49*(10), 4039–4052. https://doi.org/10.1007/s10803-019-04121-x

Cacioppo, S., Grippo, A. J., London, S., Goossens, L., & Cacioppo, J. T. (2015). Loneliness: Clinical import and interventions. *Perspectives on Psychological Science : A Journal of the Association for Psychological Science*, *10*(2), 238–249. https://doi.org/10.1177/1745691615570616

Canavarro, M. C., Simões, M. R., Vaz Serra, A., Pereira, M., Rijo, D., Quartilho, M. J., Gameiro, S., Paredes, T., & Carona, C. (2007). Instrumento de avaliação da qualidade de vida da Organização Mundial de Saúde: WHOQOL-Bref. In M. Simões, C. Machado, M. Gonçalves, & L. Almeida (Eds.), *Avaliação psicológica: Instrumentos validados para a população portuguesa* (pp. 77–100). Quarteto Editora.

Cheung, G. W., & Rensvold, R. B. (2002). Evaluating goodness-of-fit indexes for testing measurement invariance. *Structural Equation Modeling: A Multidisciplinary Journal*, *9*(2), 233–255. https://doi.org/10.1207/S15328007SEM0902_5

Cohen, J. (1992). A power primer. *Psychological Bulletin*, *112*(1), 155–159. https://doi.org/10.1037//0033-2909.112.1.155

Cohen, J., Cohen, P., West, S., & Aiken, L. (2003). *Applied multiple regression/correlation analysis for the behavioural sciences* (3th ed.). Lawrence Erlbaum Associates.

Dong, X., Chang, E., Wong, E., & Simon, M. (2012). Perception and negative effect of loneliness in a Chicago Chinese population of older adults. *Archives of Gerontology and Geriatrics*, *54*(1), 151–159. https://doi.org/10.1016/j.archger.2011.04.022

Dowd, A. J., & Jung, M. E. (2017). Self-compassion directly and indirectly predicts dietary adherence and quality of life among adults with celiac disease. *Appetite*, *113*, 293–300. https://doi.org/10.1016/j.appet.2017.02.023

Field, A. P. (2004). *Discovering statistics using SPSS* (3rd ed.). Sage.

Finlay-Jones, A., Boyes, M., Perry, Y., Sirois, F., Lee, R., & Rees, C. (2020). Online self-compassion training to improve the well-being of youth with chronic medical conditions: Protocol for a randomised control trial. *BioMed Central Public Health*, *20*(106), 1–10. https://doi.org/10.1186/s12889-020-8226-7

Gilbert, P. (2017). *Compassion: Concepts, research and applications*. Routledge.

Gilbert, P., Catarino, F., Duarte, C., Matos, M., Kolts, R., Stubbs, J., Ceresatto, L., Duarte, J., Pinto-Gouveia, J., & Basran, J. (2017). The development of compassionate engagement and action scales for self and others. *Journal of Compassionate Health Care*, *4*(1). https://doi.org/10.1186/s40639-017-0033-3

Gilbert, P. & Choden , (2013). *Mindful compassion*. Constable & Robinson.

Hawkley, L. C., & Cacioppo, J. T. (2010). Loneliness matters: A theoretical and empirical review of consequences and mechanisms. *Annals of Behavioral Medicine : A Publication of the Society of Behavioral Medicine*, *40*(2), 218–227. https://doi.org/10.1007/s12160-010-9210-8

Hawkley, L. C., Thisted, R. A., Masi, C. M., & Cacioppo, J. T. (2010). Loneliness predicts increased blood pressure: 5-year cross-lagged analyses in middle-aged and older adults. *Psychology and Aging*, *25*(1), 132–141. https://doi.org/10.1037/a0017805

Heide, I. V., Snoeijs, S., Melchiorre, M. G., Quattrini, S., Boerma, W., Schellevis, F., & Rijken, M. (2015). *Innovating care for people with multiple chronic conditions in Europe*. Nivel.

Hermanto, N., Zuroff, D. C., Kopala-Sibley, D. C., Kelly, A. C., Matos, M., Gilbert, P., & Koestne, R. (2016). Ability to receive compassion from others buffers the depressogenic effect of self-criticism: A cross-cultural multi-study analysis. *Personality and Individual Differences*, *98*, 324–332. https://doi.org/10.1016/j.paid.2016.04.055

Hlabangana, V., & Hearn, J. H. (2020). Depression in partner caregivers of people with neurological conditions; associations with self-compassion and quality of life. *Journal of Mental Health*, *29*(2), 176–181. https://doi.org/10.1080/09638237.2019.1630724

Holt-Lunstad, J., Smith, T. B., & Layton, J. B. (2010). Social relationships and mortality risk: A meta-analytic review. *PLoS Medicine*, *7*(7), e1000316. https://doi.org/10.1371/journal.pmed.1000316

Hu, L., & Bentler, P. (1999). Cutoff criteria for fit indexes in covariance structure analysis: Conventional criteria versus new alternatives. *Structural Equation Modeling: A Multidisciplinary Journal*, *6*(1), 1–55. https://doi.org/10.1080/10705519909540118

Hyland, K. A., Small, B. J., Gray, J. E., Chiappori, A., Creelan, B. C., Tanvetyanon, T., Nelson, A. M., Cessna-Palas, J., Jim, H. S. L., & Jacobsen, P. B. (2019). Loneliness as a mediator of the relationship of social cognitive variables with depressive symptoms and quality of life in lung cancer patients beginning treatment. *Psycho-Oncology*, *28*(6), 1234–1242. https://doi.org/10.1002/pon.5072

Itzick, M., Kagan, M., & Ben-Ezra, M. (2018). Social worker characteristics associated with perceived meaning in life. *Journal of Social Work*, *18*(3), 326–347. https://doi.org/10.1177/1468017316654345

Kilian, R., Matschinger, H., & Angermeyer, M. C. (2001). The impact of chronic illness on subjective quality of life: A comparison between general population and hospital in patients with somatic and psychiatric diseases. *Clinical Psychology & Psychotherapy*, *8*(3), 206–213. https://doi.org/10.1002/cpp.277

Kline, R. (2005). *Principles and practice of structural equation modelling* (3rd ed.). The Guilford Press.

Leigh-Hunt, N., Bagguley, D., Bash, K., Turner, V., Turnbull, S., Valtorta, N., & Caan, W. (2017). An overview of systematic reviews on the public health consequences of social isolation and loneliness. *Public Health*, *152*, 157–171. https://doi.org/10.1016/j.puhe.2017.07.035

Lyon, T. A. (2015). Self-compassion as a predictor of loneliness: The relationship between self-evaluation processes and perceptions of social connection. *Selected Honors Theses*, *37*. http://firescholars.seu.edu/honors

McClelland, H., Evans, J. J., Nowland, R., Ferguson, E., & O'Connor, R. C. (2020). Loneliness as a predictor of suicidal ideation and behaviour: A systematic review and meta-analysis of prospective studies. *Journal of Affective Disorders, 274*, 880–896. https://doi.org/10.1016/j.jad.2020.05.004

McIntyre, E., Lauche, R., Frawley, J., Sibbritt, D., Reddy, P., & Adams, J. (2019). Physical activity and depression symptoms in women with chronic illness and the mediating role of health-related quality of life. *Journal of Affective Disorders, 252*, 294–299. https://doi.org/10.1016/j.jad.2019.04.057

Newall, N. E., Chipperfield, J. G., Clifton, R. A., Perry, R. P., Swift, A. U., & Ruthig, J. C. (2009). Causal beliefs, social participation, and loneliness among older adults: A longitudinal study. *Journal of Social and Personal Relationships, 26*(2–3), 273–290. https://doi.org/10.1177/0265407509106718

Niccoli, T., & Partridge, L. (2012). Ageing as a risk factor for disease. *Current Biology : Cb, 22*(17), R741–752. https://doi.org/10.1016/j.cub.2012.07.024

O'Halloran, J., Miller, G. C., & Britt, H. (2004). Defining chronic conditions for primary care with ICPC-2. *Family Practice, 21*(4), 381–386. https://doi.org/10.1093/fampra/cmh407

Özkan Tuncay, F., Fertelli, T., & Mollaoğlu, M. (2018). Effects of loneliness on illness perception in persons with a chronic disease. *Journal of Clinical Nursing, 27*(7–8), e1494–1500. https://doi.org/10.1111/jocn.14273

Perlman, D., & Peplau, L. A. (1982). Loneliness research: A survey of empirical findings. In L. A. Peplau & S. E. Goldston (Eds.), *Preventing the harmful consequences of severe and persistent loneliness* (pp. 13–46). National Institute of Mental Health.

Pinto-Gouveia, J., Duarte, C., Matos, M., & Fráguas, S. (2014, July–August). The protective role of self-compassion in relation to psychopathology symptoms and quality of life in chronic and in cancer patients. *Clinical Psychology & Psychotherapy, 21*(4), 311–323. https://doi.org/10.1002/cpp.1838

Pressman, S. D., Cohen, S., Miller, G. E., Barkin, A., Rabin, B. S., & Treanor, J. J. (2005). Loneliness, social network size, and immune response to influenza vaccination in college freshmen. *Health Psychology : Official Journal of the Division of Health Psychology, American Psychological Association, 24*(3), 297–306. https://doi.org/10.1037/0278-6133.24.3.297

Ribeiro, J. P., Costa, N., Vazão, M. J., Abreu, M., Pedro, L., & Silva, I. (2017). O estigma e as doenças crónicas - como o avaliar. *Psicologia, Saúde & Doença, 18*(3), 625–639. https://doi.org/10.15309/17psd180301

Rokach, A. (2012). Loneliness updated: An introduction. *The Journal of Psychology, 146*(1–2), 1–6. https://doi.org/10.1080/00223980.2012.629501

Romana, G. Q., Kislaya, I., Salvador, M. R., Gonçalves, S. C., Nunes, B., & Dias, C. (2019). Multimorbilidade em Portugal: Dados do primeiro inquérito nacional de saúde com exame físico. *Revista Científica da Ordem Dos Médicos, 32*(1), 30–37. https://doi.org/10.20344/amp.11227

Russell, D. (1996). UCLA Loneliness Scale (Version 3): Reliability, validity, and factor structure. *Journal of Personality Assessment, 66*(1), 20–40. https://www.iscet.pt/sites/default/files/imce/ucla_loneliness_scale_version_3._reliability_validity_and_factor_structure.pdf

Russell, D. W., Cutrona, C. E., McRae, C., & Gomez, M. (2012). Is Loneliness the Same as Being Alone?*The Journal of Psychology, 146*(1–2), 7–22. https://doi.org/10.1080/00223980.2011.589414

Russell, D., Cutrona, C. E., Rose, J., & Yurko, K. (1984). Social and emotional loneliness: An examination of Weiss's typology of loneliness. *Journal of Personality and Social Psychology, 46*(6), 1313–1321. https://doi.org/10.1037/0022-3514.46.6.1313

Schrempft, S., Jackowska, M., Hamer, M., & Steptoe, A. (2019). Associations between social isolation, loneliness, and objective physical activity in older men and women. *BioMed Central Public Health, 19*(74). http://doi.org/10.1186/s12889-019-6424-y

Shovestul, B., Han, J., Germine, L., & Dodell-Feder, D. (2020). Risk factors for loneliness: The high relative importance of age versus other factors. *PLoS One, 15*(2), e0229087. https://doi.org/http://doi.org/10.31234/osf.io/t8n2h

Sirois, F. M., & Hirsch, J. K. (2019). Self-compassion and adherence in five medical samples: The role of stress. *Mindfulness, 10*(1), 46–54. https://doi.org/10.1007/s12671-018-0945-9

Stickley, A., & Koyanagi, A. (2018). Physical multimorbidity and loneliness: A population-based study. *PLoS One*, *13*(1), e0191651. https://doi.org/10.1371/journal.pone.0191651

Stickley, A., Koyanagi, A., Leinsalu, M., Ferlander, S., Sabawoon, W., & McKee, M. (2015). Loneliness and health in Eastern Europe: Findings from Moscow, Russia. *Public Health*, *129*(4), 403–410. https://doi.org/10.1016/j.puhe.2014.12.021

Tan, S. S., Fierloos, I. N., Zhang, X., Koppelaar, E., Alhambra-Borras, T., Rentoumis, T., Williams, G., Rukavina, T., Staveren, R. V., Garces-Ferrer, J., Franse, C. B., & Raat, H. (2020). The association between loneliness and health related quality of life (HR-QoL) among community-dwelling older citizens. *International Journal of Environmental Research and Public Health*, *17*(2), 6001–6012. https://doi.org/10.3390/ijerph17020600

Trindade, I. A., Duarte, J., Ferreira, C., Coutinho, M., & Pinto-Gouveia, J. (2018). The impact of illness-related shame on psychological health and social relationships: Testing a mediational model in students with chronic illness. *Clinical Psychology & Psychotherapy*, *25*(3), 408–414. https://doi.org/10.1002/cpp.2175

Ward, B. W., & Schiller, J. S. (2013). Prevalence of multiple chronic conditions among US adults: Estimates from the National Health Interview Survey, 2010. *Preventing Chronic Disease*, *10*, E65. https://doi.org/10.5888/pcd10.120203

WHOQOL Group. (1994). Development of the WHOQOL: Rationale and current status. *International Journal of Mental Health*, *23*(3), 24–56. https://doi.org/10.1080/00207411.1994.11449286

WHOQOL Group. (1998). Development of the World Health Organization WHOQOL-BREF quality of life assessment. *Psychological Medicine*, *28*, 551–558. https://doi.org/10.5.12

Wollast, R., Riemer, A. R., Bernard, P., Leys, C., Kotsou, I., & Klein, O. (2019). How self-compassion moderates the effect of body surveillance on subjective happiness and depression among women. *Scandinavian Journal of Psychology*, *60*(5), 464–472. https://doi.org/10.1111/sjop.12553

Zeas-Sigüenza, A., Ganho, A., Ruisoto, P., & Ferreira, C. (2020). *Validation of the Portuguese version of UCLA Loneliness Scale Version- 3* [Manuscript in preparation]. Faculdade de Psicologia e Ciências da Educação, Universidade de Coimbra.

How Future Orientation is Associated with Depressive Symptoms in Multiethnoracial Adults: Basic Psychological Needs as a Mediator

Edward C. Chang, Olivia D. Chang, Elizabeth A. Yu, Kaidi Wu, Abigael G. Lucas, P. Priscilla Lui, David Rollock, Xinjie Chen, Jameson K. Hirsch and Elizabeth L. Jeglic

ABSTRACT
We examined the role of basic psychological needs as a mediator of the association between future orientation and depressive symptoms in a sample of 202 (159 female and 43 male) multiethnoracial adults. Multiple mediation analysis with 10,000 bootstraps was conducted to test for mediation. The association between future orientation and depressive symptoms was found to be accounted for by dimensions of basic psychological needs. Specifically, future orientation was negatively related to depressive symptoms through positive associations involving autonomy and competence, but not relatedness. The present findings are the first to not only point to the importance of examining future orientation in understanding depressive symptoms in multiethnoracial adults, but they are also the first to suggest possible mechanisms by which believing in a changeable future might foster stronger satisfaction of basic psychological needs, especially autonomy and competence, that might help multiethnoracials garner greater protection when encountering stressful situations in their lives.

As researchers have argued, much of what we know in psychological science remains predominantly based on the study of Western, educated, industrialized, rich and democratic (WEIRD) populations (e.g., Graham, 1992; Henrich, Heine, & Norenzayan, 2010). By 2060, it is projected that ethnoracial groups will make up more than 55% of the American population (U.S. Census Bureau, 2015). Within the current population of minority ethnoracial groups, multiethnoracials, individuals who identify with two or greater ethnoracial heritages based on their lived experience and upon conventional ethnoracial classifications (Lou & Lalonde, 2015), make up one of the smallest groups. However, multiethnoracials represent one of the fastest growing groups among all ethnoracial groups, with an estimate of more than 9.3 million Americans identifying themselves being of two or greater ethnicities/races (U. S. Census Bureau, 2016). Noteworthy, findings from studies indicate that multiethnoracials, compared to monoethnoracials, are at greater risk of substance use and violence (Choi, Harachi, Gillmore, & Catalano, 2006). Additionally, when compared to related ethnoracial minority groups, those of multiethnoracial status (e.g., multiethnoracial Hispanics compared to Hispanics) have been found to experience greater psychological and behavioral problems (e.g., substance use, depression, & risk for suicide; Whaley & Francis, 2006). Furthermore, findings from other studies have also pointed to the unique experience of strain associated with being "culturally homeless" that is exclusive to multiethnoracials (Navarrete & Jenkins, 2011). Accordingly, in the context of predicting important psychological outcomes, it has become a priority for researchers to identify variables associated with the psychological adjustment of a growing number of diverse ethnoracial groups, including multiethnoracials who may be at even greater risk for depression (Sanchez, Shih, & Garcia, 2009). In that regard, although strategies to predict depressive symptoms, and other negative affective conditions, have typically been based on identifying negative individual differences variables, there may be value in considering positive individual differences variables as well (Chang, Downey, Hirsch, & Lin, 2016).

Positive future cognitions represent a potentially important category of variables for understanding psychological adjustment in adults (Wingate et al., 2006). In contrast to general positive future cognitions that are predicated on broad and general expectations that good things will happen (e.g., optimism; Scheier & Carver, 1985), future orientation is predicated on the general belief that despite experiencing stressful situations, one's future will change for the better (e.g., stop feeling bad, reach desired goals, be engaged in effective action; Hirsch et al., 2006), which should help secure greater positive adjustment (e.g., be happier, be less sad). That is, believing that the future will be less stressful is expected to help individuals eventually feel happier or feel less sad. Indeed, findings from recent research studies have identified a reliable negative association between future orientation and depressive symptoms across different cultural populations (e.g., Americans, Hungarians; Chang, Chang, Martos, & Sallay, 2017a; Chang et al., 2017c; Chang et al., 2013). However, the examination of future orientation as a predictor of depressive symptoms has yet to be conducted in studies of minority ethnoracial groups, including multiethnoracials. Indeed, given that there appears to be some evidence to suggest that multiethnoracials may specifically experience more (not less) stress and strain associated with having to effectively navigate across multiple ethnic and racial identities compared to monoethnoracials (e.g., Sanchez et al., 2009; Whaley & Francis, 2006), an examination of the role of future orientation in multiethnoracials seemed especially warranted.

Beyond identifying an association between future orientation and depressive symptoms in multiethnoracials, it might also be important to consider motivational mechanisms that might help account for such a relationship. One theoretical variable that may be useful in accounting for the link between future orientation and depressive symptoms is the ability to meet basic psychological needs. According to Deci and Ryan's (2000, 2008) self-determination theory, the ability to meet or satisfy basic human psychological needs (viz., autonomy, competence, & relatedness) plays a critical role in determining individual differences in adjustment. Consistent with this view, findings from numerous studies have indicated that lower satisfaction of core psychological needs are positively associated with negative psychological outcomes (e.g., depressive

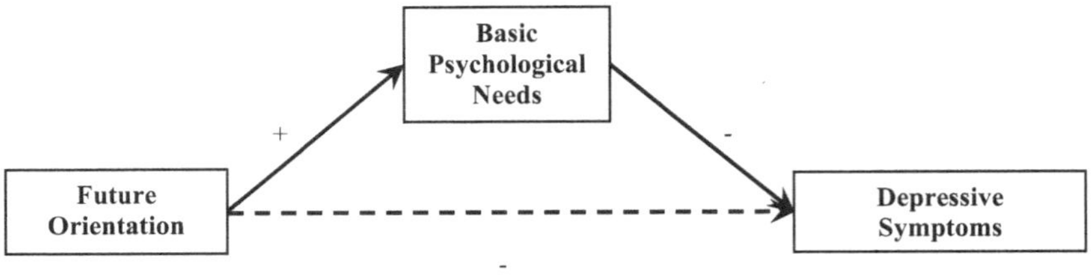

Figure 1. Hypothesized mediation model of the relationship between future orientation and depressive symptoms mediated by basic psychological needs.

symptoms; see Deci & Ryan, 2000, for a review). For example, Wei, Shaffer, Young, and Zakalik (2005) found that lower basic psychological needs satisfaction was strongly associated with greater depressive symptoms in college students. Moreover, Chang et al. (2015) found that psychological needs, in particular, autonomy and competence, mediated the positive association between sexual assault victimization and depressive symptoms in college students. In both studies, however, the adult sample was predominantly Caucasian/European American. Indeed, as noted by Luginbuhl, McWhirter, and McWhirter (2016), although self-determination theory represents a promising inclusive theory for understanding behavior, it has largely been underutilized in the study of minority ethnoracial groups. Thus, in the present study, we also sought to determine if the ability to meet basic psychological needs might mediate the association between future orientation and transient depressive symptoms in multiethnoracial adults (see Figure 1).

Purpose of the present study

Based on these considerations, the purpose of the present study was to: 1) examine the relations between future orientation, basic psychological needs, and depressive symptoms in multiethnoracial adults; and 2) determine if basic psychological needs (viz., autonomy, competence, and relatedness) might account for the expected association to be found between future orientation and depressive symptoms in multiethnoracial adults.

Consistent with past research findings (e.g., Chang et al., 2017a; Chang et al., 2017c; Chang et al., 2013), we expected future orientation to be negatively correlated with depressive symptoms. Similarly, given Deci and Ryan's (2000) theory of basic psychological needs and past research findings linking basic psychological needs with lower risk of maladjustment, we expected these core psychological needs to be associated with lower depressive symptoms. Furthermore, consistent with the notion that positive cognitions can often help activate behavior towards goal achievement, we expected future orientation to be associated with higher satisfaction of basic psychological needs.

Finally, consistent with our hypothesized mediation model, we expected to find evidence consistent with the notion that the negative association between future orientation and depressive symptoms would be fully accounted for by the ability to satisfy basic psychological needs. Given the lack of studies conducted on minority ethnoracial groups, we expected each basic psychological needs dimension to represent an important mediator of the link between future orientation and depressive symptoms.

Method

Participants

A total of 202 college students (159 females and 43 males) who indicated having two or greater ethnoracial identities (e.g., "Black, not of Hispanic origin", "Hispanic," "Caucasian," "American Indian or Alaska Native," and "Asian or Pacific Islander") were recruited from a large Eastern public university in the United States. Ages ranged from 18 to 39 years, with a mean age of 20.57 ($SD = 3.34$).

Measures

Future orientation

Future orientation was assessed by the Future Orientation Scale (FOS; Hirsch et al., 2006). The FOS is a 6-item self-report measure that was developed to assess for an individual's belief and appreciation that the future would be changed even when experiencing stressful circumstances or negative events (e.g., "No matter how badly I feel, I know it will not last"). Respondents are asked to indicate "how important each reason is to you for dealing with stressors" using a 5-point Likert-type scale, ranging from 1 (*extremely unimportant*) to 5 (*extremely important*). In general, higher scores on the FOS indicate a greater belief that one's future can be changed for the better. In the present sample, internal consistency of the FOS as measured by Cronbach α was .90.

Basic psychological needs

To assess for basic psychological needs, we used the General Basic Psychological Needs Scale (GBPNS; Gagné, 2003). The GBPNS is a 21-item self-report measure and consists of three separate subscales, namely, autonomy (e.g., "I feel like I am free to decide for myself how to live my life"), competence (e.g., "People I know tell me I am good at what I do"), and relatedness (e.g., "I get along with people I come into contact with"). Participants are asked to respond to each item on a 7-point Likert-type scale, ranging from 1 (*not at all true*) to 7 (*very true*), regarding how well each psychological need is generally satisfied in their life. Higher scores on the GBPNS subscales indicate greater needs satisfaction. In the present sample, internal consistencies of the GBPNS subscales as measured by Cronbach α ranged from .76 (Autonomy) to .81 (Relatedness).

Depressive symptoms

To assess for depressive symptoms, we used the Beck Depression Inventory (BDI; Beck, Ward, Mendelson, Mock, & Erbaugh, 1961). The BDI is a commonly used 21-item self-report measure of depressive symptomatology. Respondents are asked to rate the extent to which they have experienced specific depressive symptoms in the past week, across a 4-point Likert-type scale (e.g. "0 = *I do not feel sad*" to "3 = *I am so sad or unhappy that I can't stand it*"). In support for construct validity, Beck et al. (1961) found that scores on the BDI were positively associated with scores on other measures of depressive symptoms and with clinical ratings of depression. Higher scores on the BDI indicate

Table 1. Descriptive Statistics for the Present Multiethnoracial Adult Sample.

	n	%
Gender		
Male	43	21.3%
Female	159	78.7%
Age		
25 or younger	185	91.6%
Older than 25 yr	17	8.4%
Class breakdown		
Freshman	76	37.6%
Sophomore	48	23.8%
Junior	51	25.2%
Senior	27	13.4%
Annual family income		
Less than $10,000	36	17.7%
$10,000–$20,000	44	21.7%
$20,000–$30,000	30	14.8%
$30,000–$40,000	18	8.9%
$40,000–$50,000	14	6.9%
$50,000–$60,000	16	7.9%
$60,000–$70,000	14	6.9%
$70,000–$80,000	8	3.9%
Greater than $80,000	23	11.3%
Immigration status		
Did not immigrate to US	186	92.1%
Did immigrate to US	16	7.9%

Note. $n = 202$.

greater depressive symptoms. In the present sample, internal consistency of the BDI as measured by Cronbach α was .93.

Procedure

Self-identified multiethnoracial college students taking an Introduction to Psychology course were solicited to participate in a paper-and-pencil study looking at personality and adjustment using a Psychology Subject Pool website. A total of 202 multiethnoracials signed up for the study online and then completed all study measures a few days later in a group setting. The study included a self-report battery involving the FOS, GBPNS, BDI, and several sociodemographic questions (e.g., age, sex, family income). Measures were randomized to control for ordering effects. The battery was administered in groups of 15 participants or greater. Participants were not made aware of the purpose of the study until after the study was completed. Upon completion, students were given research credit for their participation. All participants signed consent forms and were informed that all test data would be kept strictly confidential.

Results

As shown in Table 1, the majority of the multiethnoracial participants were female (78.7%), aged $\leq$ 25 years (91.6%), freshman (37.6%), born in the US (92.1%), and over half (54.2%) reported annual household incomes $\leq$ $30,000. As Table 2 shows, the majority of the multiethnoracial participants reported "Hispanic" ($n = 161$) as one of their multiethnoracial identities (79.7%). Of the 80 participants who indicated "Hispanic/Other," these typically involved responses in which participants identified

Table 2. Self-Identified Ethnoracial Breakdown of the Present Multiethnoracial Adult Sample.

	n	%
Ethnoracial group		
Asian, Other	2	1.0%
Black, Asian	3	1.5%
Black, Caucasian	11	5.4%
Black, Caucasian, Indian	1	0.5%
Black, Hispanic	24	11.9%
Black, Hispanic, Caucasian	1	0.5%
Black, Hispanic, Caucasian, Indian	2	1.0%
Black, Hispanic, Caucasian, Indian, Asian, Other	1	0.5%
Black, Hispanic, Caucasian, Other	1	0.5%
Black, Hispanic, Indian	1	0.5%
Black, Indian	3	1.5%
Black, Other	5	2.5%
Caucasian, Asian	7	3.5%
Caucasian, Indian	4	2.0%
Caucasian, Other	4	2.0%
Hispanic, Asian	8	4.0%
Hispanic, Asian, Other	1	0.5%
Hispanic, Caucasian	34	16.8%
Hispanic, Caucasian, Asian	1	0.5%
Hispanic, Caucasian, Other	4	2.0%
Hispanic, Indian	2	1.0%
Hispanic, Indian, Other	1	0.5%
Hispanic, Other	80	39.6%

Note. $n = 202$.

more than one Hispanic country of origin, with the most common combination reported being "Puerto Rican" and "Dominican".

Relations between future orientation, basic psychological needs, and depressive symptoms in multiethnoracial adults

Correlations between all measures are presented in Table 3. As this table shows, the patterns of correlations were generally consistent with expectations. For example, FOS scores were positively correlated with scores on the GBPNS subscales ($rs = .37$ to .43, $ps < .001$) and negatively correlated with scores on the BDI ($r = -.26$, $p < .001$). Similarly, scores on the three GBPNS subscales were found to be negatively correlated with scores on the BDI ($rs = -.47$ to $-.56$, $ps < .001$).

Examining basic psychological needs as a potential mediator of the link between future orientation and depressive symptoms in multiethnoracial adults

To examine for the potential role of each of the three basic psychological needs dimensions as potential mediators, we tested a hypothesized multiple mediation model, involving autonomy, competence, and relatedness as potential mediators of the link between future orientation and depressive symptoms. We used Preacher and Hayes' (2008) bootstrapping methods for detecting total indirect effects and specific indirect effects when multiple mediators are involved in the prediction model. Bootstrapping with 10,000 resamples was used to obtain parameter estimates for both total and specific indirect effects. If the 95% bias-corrected confidence interval does not contain a zero, then the

Table 3. Correlations, Means, Standard Deviations, and Internal Reliability Estimates for All Study Variables.

Variables	1	2	3	4	5
Future orientation	–	–	–	–	–
Autonomy	0.43***	–	–	–	–
Competence	0.37***	0.73***	–	–	–
Relatedness	0.38***	0.67***	0.65***	–	–
Depressive symptoms	−0.26***	−0.56***	−0.55***	−0.47***	–
M	29.79	35.00	30.79	42.50	11.01
SD	6.33	7.29	6.44	8.12	9.93

Notes. $n = 202$.
***$p < .001$.

Table 4. Indirect Effects of Future Orientation by Autonomy, Competence, and Relatedness on Depressive Symptoms in Multiethnoracial Adults.

Mediator	Parameter estimate	*SE*	95% BC CI	
			Lower	Upper
Depressive symptoms				
Total	−0.41	0.09	−0.61	−0.25*
Autonomy	−0.20	0.09	−0.42	−0.05*
Competence	−0.15	0.06	−0.30	−0.05*
Relatedness	−0.06	0.05	−0.19	0.03
C1	−0.05	0.13	−0.32	0.18
C2	−0.14	0.12	−0.42	0.05
C3	−0.09	0.08	−0.27	0.05

Notes. $n = 202$. C1 = Pairwise contrast for autonomy and competence; C2 = pairwise contrast for autonomy and relatedness; C3 = pairwise contrast for competence and relatedness; BC CI = bias-corrected confidence interval.
*$p < .05$.

indirect effect is considered statistically significant and mediation is demonstrated (Preacher & Hayes, 2008).

Results of computing parameter estimates for detecting total and specific indirect effects on the relation between future orientation and depressive symptoms as mediated by autonomy, competence, and relatedness are presented in Table 4. As the table shows, the total indirect effect, as well as the specific indirect effects of autonomy and competence, were found to be significant ($p < .05$). Interestingly, the specific indirect effect involving relatedness as a mediator of the link between future orientation and depressive symptoms was not found to be significant. As shown in Figure 2, the hypothesized effects of mediation for both autonomy and competence were full, as autonomy and competence were significantly and positively related to future orientation (*B*s = .49 and .37, respectively), as well as significantly and negatively related to depressive symptoms (*B*s = –.40 and –.41, respectively). As noted above, the indirect effect involving relatedness was not found to be significant. Although the association between future orientation and relatedness was significant and positive ($B = .50$), the association between relatedness and depressive symptoms was not significant ($B = -.12$). Finally, the results of conducting a pairwise contrast of indirect effects revealed that the specific indirect effect of autonomy was not stronger than that of competence. The overall model involving future orientation and basic psychological needs was found to account for a large ($f^2 = .57$) 36.2% of the variance in depressive symptoms, $F(4, 197) = 31.38$, $p < .001$.

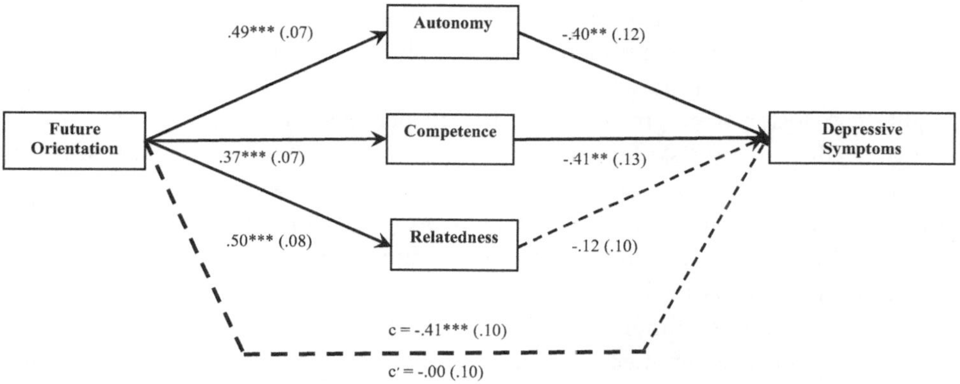

Figure 2. A multiple mediation model of the relationship between future orientation and depressive symptoms mediated by autonomy, competence, and relatedness. All numbers are nonstandardized regression coefficients and their standard errors.

Discussion

Given the lack of studies examining positive psychological constructs that are related to psychological adjustment in minority ethnoracial groups (Chang et al., 2016; Wingate et al., 2006), we conducted the present study to examine the relationship between future orientation, basic psychological needs, and depressive symptoms in multiethnoracial adults. Overall, our correlational findings were consistent with those from past studies based on non-minority ethnoracial groups (e.g., Chang et al., 2013; Hirsch et al., 2006). For example, we found that future orientation was associated with higher satisfaction of all three basic psychological needs, and with lower levels of depressive symptoms. Thus, multiethnoracials who believed that their future would change for the better, even when experiencing stressful situations, were more inclined to see themselves as independent, capable, and interpersonally relatable, and less inclined to experience depressive symptoms.

Basic psychological needs as a mediator of the link between future orientation and depressive symptoms in multiethnoracial adults

As discussed earlier, although a negative association between future orientation and depressive symptoms has been reliably identified in past studies based largely on non-minority ethnoracial groups (e.g., Chang et al., 2017a; Chang et al., 2017c; Chang et al., 2013), little work has been done to examine for mechanisms that might account for this important relationship. Based on Deci and Ryan's (2000, 2008) contention that basic psychological needs play a central role in psychological adjustment, we tested a hypothetical mediation model in which the expected negative association to be found between future orientation and depressive symptoms in multiethnoracials might be accounted for by one's ability to satisfy their basic psychological needs. Consistent with our hypothesized model, we found support for mediation involving two of the three basic psychological needs. Specifically, autonomy and competence, but not relatedness, were found to mediate the previously significant association between future orientation and depressive symptoms in multiethnoracials. Thus, our findings are consistent with the notion that for multiethnoracials, believing that the future would change for the better might help foster their greater sense of independence and competence, which in turn might reduce their risk for experiencing depressive symptoms. That said, given that Chang et al. (2015) also found autonomy and competence, but not relatedness, to represent unique proximal determinants of depressive symptoms in a predominantly White sample of adults, it may be that these two dimensions of psychological needs represent common pathways to the development of depression and other negative affective conditions across diverse ethnoracial groups. Clearly, more research is not only needed to examine for the present mediation model in other ethnoracial groups (Luginbuhl et al., 2016), but also studies that examine for other negative affective conditions in adults (e.g., stress, anxiety, and suicide risk).

Overall, going beyond past studies that have primarily been limited to the study of WEIRD populations (e.g., Whites), our findings add to some emerging studies highlighting the value of applying self-determination theory to the study of psychological adjustment in minority ethnoracial groups (Luginbuhl et al., 2016). In addition, our findings suggest some possible implications for practice. Specifically, our findings suggest that in addition to carefully considering meaningful therapeutic approaches when working with multiethnoracial adults experiencing distress (Pedrotti, Edward, & Lopez, 2008), strategies to help multiethnoracials develop a strong sense of future orientation when dealing with difficult or stressful situations (e.g., ethnoracial discrimination) might especially work best in combating risk for depressive symptoms if such interventions lead to establishing a greater sense of autonomy and competence. Finally, although more research is needed, our finding that relatedness did not mediate the association between future orientation and depressive symptoms might point to the inherent challenges multiethnoracial adults typically experience when trying to be relatable to others, especially in the context of monoethnoracial adults (Remedios & Chasteen, 2013).

Some limitations of the present study

Despite these promising findings pointing to the importance of future orientation and basic psychological needs for understanding psychological adjustment in multiethnoracial adults, it is important to note some limitations. First, given our focus on young adults (i.e., college students), it remains unclear if satisfaction of basic psychological needs represents an important mediator of the link between future orientation and depressive symptoms in different adult populations (e.g., older multiethnoracials). Second, basic psychological needs satisfaction has also been linked to positive psychological outcomes in adults. Thus, for example, it would be interesting to determine if our hypothesized mediation model might be useful for predicting subjective well-being (e.g., life satisfaction, positive mood) in multiethnoracials. Third, given that the present sample was based on multiethnoracials predominantly of Hispanic identity, it would be important to determine if similar findings would emerge in a multiethnoracial sample of adults predominantly of non-Hispanic identity (e.g., Asian American, African American). For example, it would be important to determine if more specific models emerge when studying multiethoracial groups that are predominantly of a different identity (e.g., Asian "hapas" from Hawai'i). Indeed, given that Yu and Chang (2016) found future orientation held a weaker association with suicide ideation in Asians, compared to in Hispanics, it may be that the present model is less useful in studying multiethnoracials that are predominantly of Asian identity. Relatedly, it may be useful to determine if the present findings might differ when studying monoethnoracial minority groups (e.g., Hispanics). Fourth, although we focused on one important positive future cognition, namely, future orientation, it would be useful to determine if similar findings might emerge when investigating other positive future cognitions (e.g., optimism and hope; Chang et al., 2017b). Lastly, although the present study examined a hypothesized mediation model in which the positive impact of future orientation on transient depressive symptoms was expected to be accounted for by increasing one's ability to satisfy basic psychological needs in multiethnoracials, it is impossible to draw causal inferences given the cross-sectional nature of the present study. For example, it is possible that transient depressive symptoms might impact the development of resilient dispositions by decreasing one's ability to meet basic psychological needs. Therefore, it would be useful in future studies to conduct longitudinal studies to determine if future orientation in multiethnoracials is prospectively associated with increases in basic psychological needs satisfaction, which in turn is associated with decreases in depressive symptoms across time.

Concluding thoughts

Overall, the present findings are the first to not only implicate the usefulness of future orientation, a resilient positive future cognition, in understanding depressive symptoms in multiethnoracial adults, but they are also the first to suggest possible mechanisms by which believing in a changeable future might foster stronger satisfaction with dimensions of basic psychological needs, especially autonomy and competence, that are likely to help multiethnoracials garner greater protection when encountering stressful situations in their lives. In conclusion, we believe that our study offers an important first step in supporting greater efforts to promote inclusivity when applying psychological science to the study of human behavior by focusing on a very important, but much neglected population.

Acknowledgments

The first author thanks Chang Suk-Choon and Tae Myung-Sook for their encouragement and support throughout this project.

References

Beck, A. T., Ward, C. H., Mendelson, M., Mock, L., & Erbaugh, J. (1961). An inventory for measuring depression. *Archives of General Psychiatry*, *4*(6), 561–571.

Chang, E. C., Chang, O. D., Martos, T., & Sallay, V. (2017a). Future orientation and suicide risk in Hungarian college students: Burdensomeness and belongingness as mediators. *Death Studies*, *41*(5), 284–290.

Chang, E. C., Downey, C. A., Hirsch, J. K., & Lin, N. J. (2016). Introduction to positive psychology in racial and ethnic groups: A second call to action! In E. C. Chang, C. A. Downey, J. K. Hirsch, & N. J. Lin (Eds.), *Positive psychology in racial and ethnic groups: Theory, research, and practice* (pp. 3–12). Washington, DC: American Psychological Association.

Chang, E. C., Lin, J., Fowler, E. E., Yu, E. A., Yu, T., Jilani, Z., … Hirsch, J. K. (2015). Sexual assault and depressive symptoms in college students: Do psychological needs account for the relationship? *Social Work*, *60*(3), 211–218.

Chang, E. C., Martos, T., Sallay, V., Chang, O. D., Wright, K. M., Najarian, A. S.-M., & Lee, J. (2017b). Examining optimism and hope as protective factors of suicide risk in Hungarian college students: Is risk highest for those lacking positive psychological protection? *Cognitive Therapy and Research*, *41*(2), 278–288.

Chang, E. C., Wan, L., Li, P., Guo, Y., He, H., Gu, Y., … Hirsch, J. K. (2017c). Loneliness and suicidal risk in young adults: Does believing in a changeable future help minimize suicidal risk among the lonely? *The Journal of Psychology: Interdisciplinary and Applied*, *151*(5), 453–463.

Chang, E. C., Yu, E. A., Lee, J. Y., Hirsch, J. K., Kupfermann, Y., & Kahle, E. R. (2013). An examination of optimism/pessimism and suicide risk in primary care patients: Does belief in a changeable future make a difference? *Cognitive Therapy and Research*, *37*(4), 796–804.

Choi, Y., Harachi, T. W., Gillmore, M. R., & Catalano, R. F. (2006). Are multiracial adolescents at greater risk? Comparisons of rates, patterns, and correlates of substance use and violence between monoracial and multiracial adolescents. *American Journal of Orthopsychiatry*, *76*(1), 86–97.

Deci, E. L., & Ryan, R. M. (2000). The "what" and "why" of goal pursuits: Human needs and the self-determination of behavior. *Psychological Inquiry*, *11*(4), 227–268.

Deci, E. L., & Ryan, R. M. (2008). Facilitating optimal motivation and psychological well-being across life's domains. *Canadian Psychology*, *49*(1), 14–23.

Gagné, M. (2003). The role of autonomy support and autonomy orientation in prosocial behavior engagement. *Motivation and Emotion*, *27*, 199–223.

Graham, S. (1992). "Most of the subjects were White and middle class": Trends in published research on African Americans in selected APA journals, 1970-1989. *American Psychologist*, *47*(5), 629–639.

Henrich, J., Heine, S. J., & Norenzayan, A. (2010). The weirdest people in the world? *The Behavioral and Brain Sciences*, *33*(2-3), 61–135.

Hirsch, J. K., Duberstein, P. R., Conner, K. R., Heisel, M. J., Beckman, A., Franus, N., & Conwell, Y. (2006). Future orientation and suicide ideation and attempts in depressed adults ages 50 and over. *American Journal of Geriatric Psychiatry*, *14*(9), 752–757.

Lou, E., & LaLonde, R. N. (2015). Signs of transcendence? A changing landscape of multiraciality in the 21st century. *International Journal of Intercultural Relations*, *45*, 85–95.

Luginbuhl, P. J., McWhirter, E. H., & McWhirter, B. T. (2016). Sociopolitical development, autonomous motivation, and education outcomes: Implications for low-income Latina/o adolescents. *Journal of Latinta/o Psychology*, *4*(1), 43–59.

Navarrete, V., & Jenkins, S. R. (2011). Cultural homelessness, multiminority status, ethnic identity development, and self esteem. *International Journal of Intercultural Relations*, *35*(6), 791–804.

Pedrotti, J. T., Edward, L. M., & Lopez, S. J. (2008). Working with multiracial clients in therapy: Bridging theory, research, and practice. *Professional Psychology: Research and Practice*, *39*(2), 192–201.

Preacher, K. J., & Hayes, A. F. (2008). Asymptotic and resampling strategies for assessing and comparing indirect effects in multiple mediator models. *Behavior Research Methods*, *40*(3), 879–891.

Remedios, J. D., & Chasteen, A. L. (2013). Finally, someone who "gets" me! Multiracial people value others' accuracy about their race. *Cultural Diversity and Ethnic Minority Psychology*, *19*(4), 453–460.

Sanchez, D. T., Shih, M., & Garcia, J. A. (2009). Juggling multiple racial identities: Malleable racial identification and psychological well-being. *Cultural Diversity and Ethnic Minority Psychology*, *15*(3), 243–254.

Scheier, M. F., & Carver, C. S. (1985). Optimism, coping, and health: Assessment and implications of generalized outcome expectancies. *Health Psychology*, *4*(3), 219–247.

U.S. Census Bureau. (2015). *Projections of the size and composition of the U.S. population: 2014 to 2060*. Washington, DC: U.S. Census Bureau News.

U.S. Census Bureau. (2016). *Selected population profile in the United States, 2016 American community survey 1-year estimates*. Retrieved from https://factfinder.census.gov/faces/tableservices/jsf/pages/productview.xhtml?pid=ACS_16_1YR_S0201&prodType=table.

Wei, M., Shaffer, P. A., Young, S. K., & Zakalik, R. A. (2005). Adult attachment, shame, depression and loneliness: The mediation role of basic psychological needs satisfaction. *Journal of Counseling Psychology*, *52*(4), 591–601.

Whaley, A. L., & Francis, K. (2006). Behavioral health in multiracial adolescents: The role of Hispanic/Latino ethnicity. *Public Health Reports*, *121*(2), 169–174.

Wingate, L. R., Burns, A. B., Gordon, K. H., Perez, M., Walker, R. L., Williams, F. M., & Joiner, T. (2006). Suicide and positive cognitions: Positive psychology applied to the understanding and treatment of suicidal behavior. In T. E. Ellis (Ed.), *Cognition and suicide: Theory, research, and therapy* (pp. 261–283). Washington, DC: American Psychological Association.

Yu, E. A., & Chang, E. C. (2016). Optimism/pessimism and future orientation as predictors of suicidal ideation: Are there ethnic differences? *Cultural Diversity and Ethnic Minority Psychology*, *22*, 572–579.

Index